PRITIKIN DIET

MASTERPIECES FOR PREDIABETES, CARDIOVASCULAR DISEASE AND REDUCTION IN CHOLESTEROL

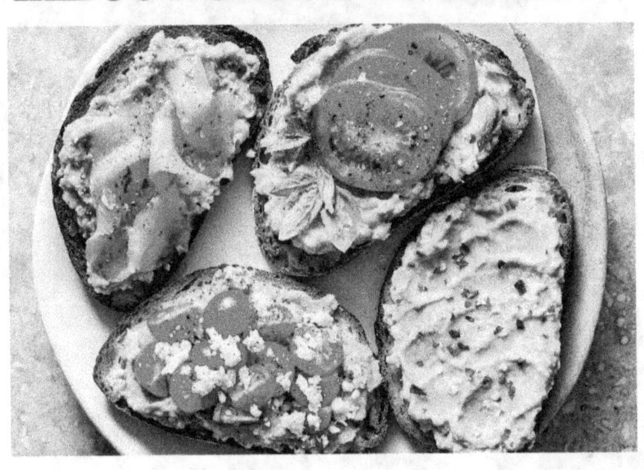

Magdalene Charles

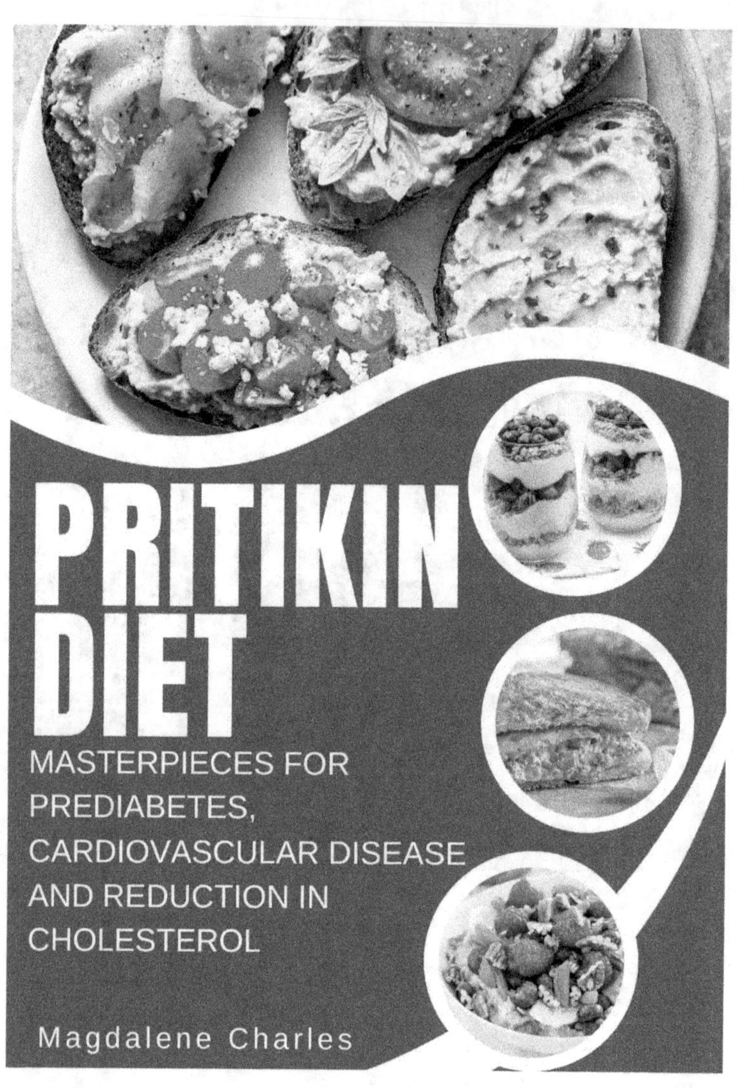
PRITIKIN
DIET
MASTERPIECES FOR
PREDIABETES,
CARDIOVASCULAR DISEASE
AND REDUCTION IN
CHOLESTEROL
Magdalene Charles

TABLE OF CONTENT

INTRODUCTION

"PRITIKIN DIET: 2024 Pritikin's Masterpieces for Prediabetes, Cardiovascular Disease, and Reduction in Cholesterol"

A thorough and practical approach to health and nutrition is more important than ever in a time when fast food, convenience, and sedentary lifestyles frequently rule our daily lives. Unprecedented obstacles to human health have emerged in the twenty-first century, including the ongoing problem of high cholesterol and the increasing incidence of chronic conditions like prediabetes and cardiovascular disease.

The "PRITIKIN DIET: 2024 Pritikin's Masterpieces for Prediabetes, Cardiovascular Disease, and Reduction in Cholesterol" is a monument to the lasting strength of evidence-based nutrition and a ray of hope in this regard. Since its creation by the brilliant Nathan Pritikin several decades ago, the Pritikin Diet has undergone constant modification to reflect advancements in nutritional research and health. As of right now, it is a tried-and-true, priceless tool for anyone looking to control or avoid illnesses like excessive cholesterol, cardiovascular disease, and prediabetes.

This book is a tribute to Pritikin's legacy, which has grown and survived the years, and it offers you the most recent information, delectable recipes, and techniques to improve your general well-being in addition to your health. Through "PRITIKIN DIET: 2024 Pritikin's Masterpieces," you will learn how the Pritikin principles have been updated and refined to solve the particular health issues that plague us in this day and age.

The Pritikin Diet promotes a whole-foods-based, balanced approach to nutrition and is more than just a set of eating guidelines. It provides a long-term, healthy way to get healthier without relying on crash diets or band-aid solutions. Rather, it equips people with the information and resources they need to modify their everyday routines in a way that is both significant and long-lasting.

This book is your in-depth resource for comprehending the fundamental ideas of the Pritikin Diet, the research underlying it, and practical application strategies. It offers an abundance of delicious recipes that are adapted to suit a wide range of palates and dietary requirements, so you're never left feeling cheated or limited in your cooking options. These recipes aren't simply a list; they're thoughtfully created meals that will fuel your body and help you on your path to improved health.

You will discover a plethora of knowledge on nutrition and wellness as you peruse the pages that follow, along with the inspiration and drive to take charge of your own health. The numerous and motivational success stories of the Pritikin Diet attest to the efficacy of this strategy in changing people's lives.

Thus, the "PRITIKIN DIET: 2024 Pritikin's Masterpieces" is your reliable ally on the road to improved health, regardless of whether you have prediabetes, are worried about your cardiovascular health, or want to reduce your cholesterol. Joining us on this journey will allow you to embrace the tried-and-true Pritikin Diet's wisdom and open the door to a happier, healthier, and more vibrant version of yourself.

The path to ideal health, steered by the Pritikin Diet, is a shared one. Within these pages, you will join a thriving and constantly expanding group of people who share your objectives, difficulties, and dreams. On your journey to wellness, the community's support and friendship can serve as a source of motivation and encouragement. We may encourage one another during difficult times, exchange success stories, and rejoice in little successes.

"PRITIKIN DIET: 2024 Pritikin's Masterpieces" is a guidebook that will help you live a healthier life in the future. We will dissect complicated medical ideas into simple language as we examine the nuances of prediabetes, cardiovascular disease, and cholesterol control. You'll learn the science underlying the Pritikin Diet and be better equipped to make health-related decisions. You will realize that controlling these problems doesn't have to be a difficult or constricting task, and you will understand how the foods you eat can have a significant impact on your health.

Furthermore, this book recognizes that health is more than just what's on your plate and is based on a holistic approach to health. It discusses the value of exercise, how to handle stress, and the effectiveness of positive thinking—all of which are central tenets of the Pritikin philosophy. Together, we will investigate ways to incorporate these elements into your day-to-day activities, establishing a balanced, harmonious environment that supports your overall health.

By following the advice in "PRITIKIN DIET: 2024 Pritikin's Masterpieces," you can make decisions today that can improve your futures. Improving your health can be a lifelong gift that increases your vitality, energy, and lifespan. The possibilities are endless as you embark on your road to becoming a better, happier version of yourself.

Together, let's embrace the knowledge of Nathan Pritikin's seminal research as well as the most recent developments in nutrition and wellness as we set out on our journey. You are unlocking the door to a future that is more colorful and brighter as you turn the pages of this book. Welcome to the universe of the "PRITIKIN DIET: 2024 Pritikin's Masterpieces for Prediabetes, Cardiovascular Disease, and Reduction in Cholesterol." You're about to enter a world of vibrant health and delectable culinary creations.

As we delve further into "PRITIKIN DIET: 2024 Pritikin's Masterpieces," you'll discover that this book is a partner in your pursuit of a happier, better life, not merely a repository of knowledge. We recognize that altering your diet and way of life significantly can be difficult, but the trip is worthwhile. We've included meal plans, professional guidance, and helpful hints to help you incorporate the Pritikin principles into your everyday routine with ease. We're here to support you every step of the way.

The Pritikin Diet is based on the idea that a healthy body is the cornerstone of a happy existence. You can take proactive measures to address the growing number of health issues in today's world by implementing the ideas presented in this book. A healthy lifestyle and dietary adjustments can help manage and possibly reverse prediabetes, a condition that has the potential to develop into full-blown diabetes. Cardiovascular disease is a major global cause of death, but it can be lessened with regular exercise and a heart-healthy diet. The decisions you make in the kitchen can dramatically reduce high cholesterol, a risk factor for heart disease.

Adopting the Pritikin Diet can have a significant positive effect on your general wellbeing in addition to its health benefits. You'll experience better mood, more energy, and mental clarity. You will have a stronger immune system, which will increase your resistance to disease. Additionally, when you lose extra weight, your body image and self-confidence will improve, which is well-deserved. It's a metamorphosis that goes much beyond scale readings or lab results; it's about taking back your energy and making sure you can fully enjoy the moments in life.

We will explore the fundamental ideas of the Pritikin Diet in the upcoming chapters, including the emphasis on complete, unprocessed meals, the value of fiber, and the avoidance of added sweets and excessive salt. Additionally, you'll discover how to interpret nutrition labels and shop smarter at the grocery store. We'll provide you the resources you need to organize your meals, make delectable Pritikin-approved recipes, and investigate ways to eat out without compromising your health objectives.

You'll also hear from people who have changed their life by implementing the Pritikin Diet. Their experiences serve as motivational examples of the effectiveness of this strategy in improving health and wellbeing. We hope that you will be inspired to pursue better health by their stories and find inspiration in them.

Come along with us as we set out on this adventure of wellness, health, and delicious food. The book "PRITIKIN DIET: 2024 Pritikin's Masterpieces" is your road map to improved health, and we are honored to accompany you on this transformative journey. Here is where your journey to a better, healthier self begins, one that holds the potential for a future full of color and brightness.

CHAPTER 1 : UNDERSTANDING THE PRITIKIN APPROACH

Nathan Pritikin's Legacy and His Diet

Nathan Pritikin was a trailblazing figure in the fields of nutrition and health. He is most known for creating the Pritikin Diet, which changed the way people thought about food, health, and life expectancy. Even after his ground-breaking study was published decades ago, his legacy is characterized by his dedication to encouraging healthy living through dietary modifications and exercise.

The Early Life and Health Issues of Nathan Pritikin

Chicago, Illinois, was the birthplace of Nathan Pritikin in 1915. Although he was not meant to pursue a career in nutrition and health, his personal battles with heart disease eventually brought him to that direction. Pritikin was diagnosed with significant coronary artery disease at the age of 42. This illness frequently results in heart attacks and lowers quality of life.

Given the bleak prognosis, Pritikin started looking for a cure for his ailments. He chose to take matters into his own hands and started doing in-depth study on the relationship between diet and health because he was dissatisfied with the few options that were accessible to him at the time. His adventure into the realm of nutrition and lifestyle modification began with this.

The Pritikin Diet

Pritikin's study inspired him to create a novel method of eating for health. He thought that many chronic diseases, including heart disease, could be prevented and even reversed by following a low-fat, high-fiber, plant-based diet. His nutritional advice focused mostly on fruits, vegetables, grains, and legumes and advocated a whole-foods, low-sodium, low-cholesterol diet.

Limiting animal products, particularly red meat, and processed foods heavy in sugar and saturated fats was recommended by the Pritikin Diet. Along with dietary adjustments, Pritikin's program placed a strong emphasis on regular exercise and stress reduction methods as a whole health improvement strategy.

Scientific Validation

Nathan Pritikin was not satisfied with his own experiences attesting to the benefits of his diet. He desired scientific confirmation of his methodology. He founded the Pritikin Longevity Center in California in the 1970s, offering a structured program that followed the Pritikin Diet and exercise regimen to those with a variety of health concerns, such as diabetes and heart disease.

Numerous clinical trials and scientific investigations have validated the Pritikin Diet's tenets over time. A Pritikin-style diet has been linked to a number of heart health benefits, including decreasing blood pressure, cholesterol, and a lower risk of heart disease, according to research. These results have strengthened the reputation of Nathan Pritikin and his nutritional philosophy.

Popularization and Impact

As more people grew interested in controlling their own health through dietary adjustments, the Pritikin

Diet became more well-known in the 1970s and 1980s. It was one of the first voices, long before these concepts were widely embraced in the general public, promoting a diet reduced in cholesterol and saturated fat.

Other medical professionals and nutrition researchers were impacted by Nathan Pritikin's work. His focus on a low-fat, plant-based diet was significant in influencing the dietary guidelines of numerous government agencies and health groups. Many dietary guidelines of days, such as those from the American Diabetes Association and the American Heart Association, advocate for a diet that is mostly based on the Pritikin Diet.

Legacy and Ongoing Relevance

Nathan Pritikin's contributions to the fields of nutrition and health are still relevant today. His groundbreaking research has opened the door to a deeper comprehension of the connection between nutrition and chronic illnesses, especially heart disease. His strategy of changing one's diet and exercise routine to enhance one's overall health and lifestyle continues to motivate others to make better decisions.

Although the Pritikin Diet has changed throughout time to take into account fresh research and adjust to shifting dietary trends, its fundamental ideas have not changed. It remains a useful tool for those looking to modify their diets in order to enhance their health and lower their chance of developing chronic illnesses.

Nathan Pritikin's dedication to enhancing the quality of life for people afflicted with chronic illnesses, particularly heart disease, has left a lasting legacy in the fields of nutrition and health. Our understanding of nutrition and health has been profoundly and enduringly impacted by his innovative work in creating the Pritikin Diet. Nathan Pritikin's research continues to serve as a monument to the effectiveness of lifestyle changes in enhancing longevity and well-being, even as more people become aware of the significance of a plant-based, low-fat diet in the prevention and management of chronic illnesses.

Pritikin's Core Principles

Nathan Pritikin created the Pritikin Program, a comprehensive approach to health and fitness built around a few guiding principles. These ideas cover a comprehensive strategy for enhancing general well-being, with a particular emphasis on diet, exercise, and lifestyle adjustments. Numerous people's lives have been drastically changed by the Pritikin Core Principles, which have improved their quality of life, helped them manage chronic illnesses, and improved their overall health.

1. **Nutrition Excellence:** A whole-foods-based, plant-based diet is the cornerstone of the Pritikin Program. To do this, limit your intake of processed foods, added sugars, and excess sodium while consuming a wide range of fruits, vegetables, whole grains, legumes, and lean protein sources. This eating strategy lowers the risk of chronic illnesses like diabetes, hypertension, and heart disease in addition to helping people maintain their ideal weight.

2. **Low-Fat Living:** The Pritikin method advocates for a diet heavy in complex carbs and low in fat. It has been demonstrated that putting more of an emphasis on cutting back on dietary fat will lower blood pressure, help weight loss, and lower cholesterol. It's critical to limit saturated and trans fats and ingest healthy fats in moderation.

3. **Frequent Exercise:** An essential part of the Pritikin Program is regular exercise.

Frequent physical activity raises fitness levels, aids in weight loss, and improves cardiovascular health. The program promotes a comprehensive fitness regimen that include strength training, flexibility training, and cardiovascular activity.

4. **Stress Reduction:** The effects of stress on general health can be significant. The Pritikin Program includes stress-reduction methods including mindfulness, meditation, and relaxation exercises to help people manage the rigors of everyday life and lessen the damaging consequences of long-term stress on their health.

5. **Long-Term Lifestyle Adjustments:** The Pritikin method is a long-term lifestyle adjustment rather than a diet plan. It urges people to give up short-term fixes and make long-term changes to their routines and decisions. This guarantees that the program's advantages endure and support long-term health and wellbeing.

6. **Medical Supervision:** The Pritikin Program is frequently carried out in a setting under medical supervision. Frequent medical evaluations, such as blood tests and other measurements, aid in monitoring progress and adjusting the program to each

participant's unique medical needs. This strategy guarantees each participant's safety and effectiveness in the program.

7. **Community & Support:** For those who continue with the program, the Pritikin community is an invaluable asset. People need support and companionship to stay on track and accomplish long-lasting lifestyle changes. Exercise sessions and cookery lessons are examples of group activities that generate a supportive environment that encourages success.

8. **Scientific Support:** Evidence-based procedures and scientific research serve as the cornerstones of the Pritikin Program. The program stays at the forefront of preventive medicine since the guiding principles are updated frequently to take into account the most recent research in nutrition, exercise, and health.

9. **Personalized Approach:** The Pritikin Program acknowledges that every person has different requirements and objectives, even if the fundamental concepts are still the same. As a result, the program may be customized to address certain health issues, making it appropriate for a variety of people,

including those who are managing chronic health conditions or trying to lose weight.

10. **Long-Term Health Benefits:** Improving long-term health and well-being is the ultimate aim of the Pritikin Core Principles. People who follow these guidelines can have improved physical fitness, a lower chance of developing chronic illnesses, more energy and vitality, and an all-around higher quality of life.

11. **Nutritional Education:** One of the main goals of the Pritikin Program is to teach participants about the nutritional content of various foods. It aids people in comprehending how their food choices affect their health. Participants are better able to make educated decisions about what they eat and choose healthier options on a daily basis when nutritional literacy is promoted.

12. **Holistic Wellness:** Pritikin takes into account the connections between mental, emotional, and physical health in his holistic approach. It recognizes the connection between a sound body and a sound mind. Through stress management and relaxation techniques, the program addresses mental and emotional health, guaranteeing a

comprehensive approach to complete wellness.

13. **Chronic Disease Management:** People with long-term health issues like diabetes, high blood pressure, or high cholesterol are frequently advised to take Pritikin. Through dietary and lifestyle changes, the program can help control and even reverse some of these illnesses. Individuals are guaranteed to receive the right support and treatment when under medical supervision.

14. **Weight management:** The Pritikin Program is a useful method for reaching and keeping a healthy weight, even though it isn't only focused on weight loss. Weight management objectives are naturally supported by the emphasis on whole, low-calorie-density foods and portion control, which makes it a desirable choice for people trying to lose extra weight.

15. **Culinary Skills:** Pritikin understands the importance of cooking for a healthy lifestyle. The program teaches participants how to make scrumptious, nutrient-dense meals at home by offering cooking workshops and culinary education. This makes it possible for people to take charge of their diets and

guarantees that eating healthily may be sustainable and pleasurable.

16. **Environmental Impact:** The Pritikin Program considers how dietary decisions may affect the environment. It is consistent with sustainable and environmentally friendly eating habits that lessen the burden on the planet's resources by advocating for a plant-based diet.

17. **Healthy Aging:** Pritikin's ideas are ideal for people who want to age sensibly and keep their energy levels high as they get older. The program enhances the quality of life in senior years by fostering physical fitness, mental wellness, and cardiovascular health.

18. **Preventive Health:** The Pritikin Program's emphasis on preventive health is one of its main advantages. By adhering to these fundamental ideas, people can lower their chance of contracting chronic illnesses in the first place, encouraging a pro-active attitude to lifespan and health.

Pritikin's Core Principles offers a comprehensive strategy for health and fitness that goes beyond simple weight loss. People can change their lives and strive for increased lifespan, health, and quality of life by adopting these concepts. People of various ages and backgrounds can benefit from the program's complete and scientifically supported approach to health, which places a strong emphasis on nutrition, exercise, stress management, and continuous medical monitoring.

THE EVOLUTION OF THE PRITIKIN DIET

Named after its pioneer Nathan Pritikin, the Pritikin Diet has grown to be a well-known and major dietary plan that has changed dramatically over time. It is a fascinating exploration into the fields of wellbeing, health, and nutrition. The Pritikin Diet is examined in this article along with its history, main ideas, and expansions and modifications in response to shifting dietary fads and scientific findings.

The Pritikin Diet's History

The Vision of Nathan Pritikin

The Pritikin Diet was initially presented in the 1950s by self-taught nutritionist and inventor Nathan Pritikin. Early in life, Pritikin received a heart illness diagnosis and looked for a natural, non-surgical cure for his health issues. This was the beginning of the Pritikin Diet, which was inspired by a desire for improved health on a personal level.

Foundational Ideas

The Pritikin Diet's core tenets were plant-based, high in carbohydrates, and low in fat. Pritikin thought that the secret to heart health would be to eat a diet high in fruits, vegetables, whole grains, and legumes. In addition, he promoted a large decrease in dietary fat, especially saturated fats, and emphasized complex carbohydrates as the main energy source.

Early Achievements and Difficulties

Empirical Evidence

Pritikin established the Pritikin Longevity Center in Santa Monica, California, in the 1970s, which marked the beginning of public awareness for his dietary theories. There, participants' health significantly improved as a result of Pritikin's regimen, particularly in the management of diabetes and heart disease. The potential of the diet sparked interest after these clinical achievements.

Dissidents and Debates

The Pritikin Diet was not without controversy and its detractors. A few detractors contended that the diet was excessively stringent, while others questioned the rationale behind implementing a low-fat, high-carbohydrate strategy. The scientific and medical community are still debating these criticisms.

The Pritikin Diet's Development

Verification by Science

Scientific backing for the Pritikin Diet began to accumulate as medical research progressed. Research examining the diet's effects on blood pressure, cholesterol, and weight control started to validate its efficacy in fostering heart health and averting chronic illnesses.

Modifications and Adjustments

The Pritikin Diet changed over time in response to some of the critiques leveled at it. Changes included a more balanced approach to carbohydrate intake and allowances for specific healthy fats, like those found in nuts and seeds. The emphasis no longer lies on the severe low-fat diet that was first suggested, but rather on a whole-foods, plant-based diet.

Going Beyond Cardiovascular Health

The Pritikin Diet expanded to include a holistic approach to health. It started emphasizing weight control, diabetes prevention and management, as well as general wellbeing, in addition to heart health. Its expansion increased its attractiveness to a larger group of people.

The Pritikin Diet of Today

Pritikin Center for Longevity

Currently, the Pritikin Longevity Center, located in Miami, Florida, is home to the well-known Pritikin

Diet. The facility provides all-inclusive programs that combine behavior modification, physical activity, and medical oversight with the diet. Come to learn, practice, and adopt the Pritikin way of life.

Notoriety and Power

The Pritikin Diet has a devoted fan base, and the Ornish Diet, McDougall Diet, and the larger plant-based movement are just a few of the well-known diets and lifestyles that have been impacted by its ideas. This influence has aided in raising awareness of the significance of plant-based, whole-food diets for health promotion.

Continual Study and Improvement

The Pritikin Diet is still changing as new scientific information is incorporated. It becomes a dynamic dietary approach that can respond to the most recent information and trends when it adjusts to take into account new discoveries in nutrition and health.

Since Nathan Pritikin created the Pritikin Diet in the 1950s, it has undergone significant development. From modest beginnings as a personal journey toward improved health, it has developed into a well-known and significant eating plan. The diet is still relevant and useful for promoting health and wellness in the contemporary world because it has evolved to meet the demands of practitioners, scientific research, and changing circumstances. Its evolution shows how nutrition may change people's lives and encourage a healthy future for everybody.

CHAPTER 2: PREDIABETES PREVENTION AND MANAGEMENT

Although millions of people worldwide are impacted by prediabetes, it is a serious health issue that many people may not be aware of. This disorder frequently manifests as a prelude to the onset of type 2 diabetes, a chronic illness that can be fatal. We will explore prediabetes' definition, causes, risk factors, symptoms, diagnosis, treatment options, and preventative measures in this in-depth conversation.

What Is Prediabetes?

Higher-than-normal blood sugar levels, but not high enough to be considered full-blown diabetes, are the hallmark of prediabetes. It is frequently regarded as an indicator or precursor to type 2 diabetes, a chronic illness that alters the way your body metabolizes sugar (glucose). Your blood sugar levels are increased in prediabetes, but not to the same extent as in diabetes.

Why People Get Prediabetes

Insulin resistance and insufficient pancreatic insulin synthesis are the main causes of prediabetes. Insulin is a hormone that controls blood sugar levels by making it easier for cells to use glucose as an energy source.

Blood sugar levels rise when the body loses sensitivity to the actions of insulin. Insulin resistance can be brought on by a number of things, such as bad eating habits, obesity, heredity, and physical inactivity.

Risk Elements for Type 2 Diabetes

There are certain things that can make someone more likely to get prediabetes. These consist of:

Family History: You are more likely to develop prediabetes if you have a family history of diabetes.

Obesity: Being overweight poses a serious risk, especially around the abdomen.

Passivity: Insulin resistance and prediabetes can be exacerbated by a sedentary lifestyle and insufficient physical activity.

a bad diet Prediabetes risk can be raised by diets heavy in processed and sugary foods and poor in fiber.

Age: The likelihood of developing prediabetes rises with age, especially after 45.

Ethnicity: People of African American, Hispanic American, and Native American descent are more likely to develop prediabetes.

The signs of pre-diabetes

Prediabetes is sometimes referred to be a "silent" illness because it sometimes exhibits no symptoms at all. On the other hand, some people could exhibit moderate symptoms like:

Increased Thirst: Continually experiencing thirst even after consuming liquids.

An increase in the frequency of urinating is known as frequent urination.

Fatigue: An ongoing state of exhaustion and low energy.

Vision Blur: There may be a small blurring of the vision.

Slow Wound Healing: It can take longer for cuts and sores to heal.

It's important to remember that these symptoms are not always reliable markers of prediabetes because they are frequently mild and readily confused with other conditions.

Identification of Prediabetes

Blood tests that gauge blood sugar levels are used to detect prediabetes. Among the most popular tests are:

The fasting plasma glucose test gauges your blood sugar levels following a night of fasting. 100–125 mg/dL is the range for fasting glucose levels that indicate prediabetes.

The Oral Glucose Tolerance Test (OGTT) entails an overnight fast followed by the consumption of a sweet beverage. Over the next two hours, blood sugar levels are checked at various intervals. Prediabetes is indicated by a two-hour glucose level of 140–199 mg/dL. Blood sugar levels over the previous two to three months are averaged out by the hemoglobin A1c test.

A1c values between 5.7 and 6.4% are considered prediabetic.

It's critical to act if you are diagnosed with prediabetes in order to stop or slow the onset of type 2 diabetes.

Handling and Controlling Pre-Diabetes

Lowering blood sugar levels, increasing insulin sensitivity, and lowering the risk of developing type 2 diabetes and its complications are the main objectives in managing prediabetes. The following are some methods for managing and treating prediabetes:

Lifestyle Modifications: The first line of defense against prediabetes is frequently adopting a healthy lifestyle. This entails eating a healthy, balanced diet, exercising frequently, getting rid of extra weight, and controlling stress.

Dietary modifications: Lowering blood sugar levels can be achieved by consuming fewer processed and sugary meals and raising intake of whole grains, fruits, vegetables, and lean proteins.

Physical Activity: Regular exercise helps enhance insulin sensitivity and lower blood sugar levels. Examples of this type of exercise are brisk walking, swimming, and cycling.

Drugs: To help control blood sugar levels, medical professionals may occasionally prescribe drugs. One drug that is frequently used for prediabetes is metformin.

Frequent Monitoring: People with prediabetes must regularly check their blood sugar levels and actively collaborate with medical specialists to monitor their development.

Avoidance of Pre-Diabetes

Given the risks to one's health, preventing prediabetes is not only attainable but also strongly advised. Among the preventative tactics are:

Keep a Healthy Weight: Reducing excess weight or keeping a healthy weight will help lower the chance of developing prediabetes.

Regular Physical Activity: To increase insulin sensitivity and maintain healthy blood sugar levels, aim for at least 150 minutes per week of moderate-intensity exercise.

A balanced diet should minimize processed and sugary foods and emphasize a diet high in fiber, whole grains, fruits, vegetables, and lean proteins.

Stress management: Since prolonged stress can exacerbate prediabetes, practicing stress-reduction methods like yoga or meditation can be beneficial.

Frequent Check-ups: Make an appointment for routine medical examinations to keep an eye on your general health and blood sugar levels.

prediabetes is a serious medical disorder that frequently remains undiagnosed. That is, nevertheless, a serious indicator that type 2 diabetes is developing, which can result in life-threatening health issues. Healthcare professionals and people at risk alike must comprehend the causes, risk factors, symptoms, diagnosis, and treatment of prediabetes. It is possible to delay or even stop the progression from prediabetes to full-blown diabetes and live a happier, more meaningful life by implementing lifestyle modifications and following preventative measures.

THE ROLE OF DIET IN PREDIABETES

Higher than usual blood sugar levels, but not high enough to be categorized as type 2 diabetes, are the hallmark of prediabetes. It is sometimes seen as a warning indicator, suggesting that if preventive steps are not done, there is a high probability of acquiring full-blown diabetes. A key component of managing and preventing prediabetes is diet. This thorough examination explores the complexities of nutrition and how it significantly affects prediabetes.

Recognizing Prediabetes

Prediabetes is a global disorder impacting millions of individuals. Elevated blood sugar, insulin resistance, and reduced glucose tolerance are its defining characteristics. Maintaining blood sugar control and halting the development of diabetes are essential to managing prediabetes. A key element of this method is diet.

Macronutrient Equilibrium

For people with prediabetes, maintaining a balance of macronutrients—including carbohydrates, lipids, and proteins—is essential. Blood sugar levels are most directly impacted by carbohydrates, which the body breaks down into sugar. Consequently, it is imperative to select complex carbohydrates over simple ones like white bread and refined sugar, such as whole grains, legumes, and vegetables. In order to avoid blood sugar rises, portion control is also crucial.

Intake of Fiber

A useful friend in the battle against prediabetes is dietary fiber. Whole grains, legumes, fruits, and vegetables are examples of foods high in fiber that help control blood sugar levels by slowing the absorption of sugar into the bloodstream. They also aid in satiety, which facilitates weight management—another crucial aspect of managing prediabetes.

Index of Glycemia and Load

For those who have prediabetes, knowing a food's glycemic load (GL) and glycemic index (GI) is essential. The GL considers both the amount and quality of carbohydrates in a food, while the GI gauges how rapidly a food containing carbohydrates elevates blood sugar levels. It is better to eat low-GI and GL foods since they raise blood sugar gradually and lessen the chance of spikes and crashes.

The Dietary Mediterranean

The benefits of the Mediterranean diet for prediabetes have been demonstrated by numerous studies. Whole foods including fruits, vegetables, whole grains, lean protein sources (like fish and chicken), and healthy fats (like nuts and olive oil) are prioritized in this dietary plan. It's low in sugar, processed foods, and red meat, which makes it a great option for anyone trying to control their prediabetes with diet.

Sugar and Sweetened Drinks

An important factor in the increased prevalence of prediabetes and diabetes is added sugars. Particularly, beverages with added sugar have been connected to insulin resistance and a higher chance of developing prediabetes. Reducing or eliminating sugar and sugar-containing beverages from the diet is an essential part of managing prediabetes.

Portion Regulation

Controlling portion size is essential to prediabetic management. Insulin resistance can be made worse by overeating, which can also result in weight gain and an excessive calorie intake. Blood sugar regulation can be greatly aided by practicing mindful eating and learning to identify optimal meal amounts.

Meal Schedule

The timing of snacks and meals can affect how well blood sugar is regulated. Stabilizing blood sugar levels can be achieved by eating regular, well-balanced meals and avoiding extended fasts. Smaller, more frequent meals may be helpful for some people in avoiding sugar crashes and surges.

Engagement in Exercise

Dietary measures alone are insufficient to control prediabetes. Frequent exercise is crucial for enhancing insulin sensitivity and encouraging weight loss. A healthy diet and regular exercise are two effective ways to stop prediabetes from turning into diabetes.

Tailored Dietary Plans

Since each person is different, so too can be their reaction to different foods and nutritional approaches. Consequently, customized nutrition advice—ideally from a registered dietitian or other healthcare professional—is crucial for creating a food plan that fits each person's unique requirements and interests.

A key component of managing and preventing prediabetes is diet. People with prediabetes can lower their risk of type 2 diabetes, enhance insulin sensitivity, and stabilize their blood sugar levels by adopting educated dietary decisions. It can be very beneficial to follow a well-balanced diet that has an emphasis on low-GI foods, dietary fiber, and complex carbs while limiting sugar intake. In conjunction with tailored nutrition advice and consistent physical activity, dietary tactics can enable people to take charge of their prediabetes and live longer, better lives.

BUILDING A PRITIKIN PREDIABETES PLAN

Elevated blood sugar levels outside of the diabetic range define prediabetes, a serious health condition. It is frequently seen as a warning indicator, suggesting a higher chance of getting type 2 diabetes. Thankfully, lifestyle modifications can control or even reverse prediabetes, and the Pritikin Program provides a thorough and practical method to achieve this goal. We will examine the ideas and methods of creating a Pritikin Prediabetes Plan in this extensive tutorial.

Recognizing Prediabetes

It's important to comprehend prediabetes and its consequences before beginning a Pritikin Prediabetes Plan. Blood sugar levels that are higher than usual but not high enough to be considered diabetes are referred to as prediabetes. It can develop into full-blown type 2 diabetes if untreated, which can cause serious health issues.

The Pritikin Initiative

A plant-centric, whole-foods-based approach to health and wellness is the Pritikin Program. It places a strong emphasis on managing stress, eating a diet high in whole, unprocessed foods, exercising frequently, and making significant lifestyle adjustments. The Pritikin Program is very useful when used to manage prediabetes.

Creating a Plan for Pritikin Prediabetes

Speak with a Healthcare expert: It's imperative to speak with a healthcare expert prior to starting any prediabetes management program. They are able to offer an accurate diagnosis, evaluate your unique needs, and track your advancement all the way through your journey. This advice guarantees that you get the right treatment based on your unique health situation.

Adopt a Plant-Centric Diet: A diet high in plant-based, whole foods is the cornerstone of the Pritikin Program. Key ideas consist of:

Fruits and veggies: Try to have a half-full plate of vibrant, non-starchy fruits and vegetables.

Whole grains: Refined grains should be avoided in favor of whole grains like quinoa, brown rice, and oats.

Lean proteins: Include sources of lean protein such lentils, beans, and skinless chicken.

Limit processed foods and added sugars: Cut back on or give up highly processed foods and those with a lot of added sugar.

Control Serving Sizes

Maintaining blood sugar levels requires careful attention to portion proportions. Lowering portion sizes can help control blood sugar levels and avoid overindulging. An essential first step in portion control is learning to recognize your body's hunger signals.

Exercise on a Regular Basis: Exercise is a very effective way to manage prediabetes. Aiming for at least 150 minutes of moderate-intensity aerobic exercise or 75 minutes of vigorous-intensity aerobic exercise per week, the Pritikin Program promotes regular physical activity. To increase insulin sensitivity and develop muscle, strength exercise is also crucial.

Weight management: Even a small reduction in weight can have a major positive impact on insulin sensitivity if you are overweight. The Pritikin Program promotes weight loss that is steady and gradual by combining food modifications with frequent exercise.

Check Blood Sugar Levels: As directed by your healthcare professional, check your blood sugar levels on a regular basis. You may monitor your development and make sure your prediabetes is under control with the aid of this.

Stress Reduction: Stress has an effect on blood sugar levels. To support emotional wellbeing, the

Pritikin Program promotes stress-reduction methods like mindfulness, meditation, and relaxation training.

Accountability and Support: To maintain accountability and motivation during your journey, look for assistance from medical specialists, licensed dietitians, and support groups. Having a community of support around you can have a big impact on how you manage prediabetes.

Long-Term Commitment: Managing diabetes requires a lifetime commitment to a healthy lifestyle. It is not a temporary activity. The Pritikin Program encourages long-term, sustainable behaviors that can control prediabetes and lower your chance of getting type 2 diabetes.

Managing and even reversing prediabetes with diet, exercise, stress reduction, and lifestyle modifications is possible with the help of the Building a Pritikin Prediabetes Plan. People with prediabetes can take charge of their health and lower their chance of developing type 2 diabetes by adhering to a plant-centric, whole-food diet and seeking medical advice. Accepting the tenets and techniques of the Pritikin Program will enable you to live a longer, healthier life.

CHAPTER 3: CARDIOVASCULAR DISEASE DEMYSTIFIED

CARDIOVASCULAR HEALTH AND ITS IMPORTANCE

The state of the heart and blood arteries, which comprise the cardiovascular system, is referred to as cardiovascular health. Given the critical role the cardiovascular system plays in supporting life, maintaining excellent cardiovascular health is extremely important. The heart circulates blood that is rich in oxygen to different organs and tissues, giving them the nourishment and oxygen they require to function at their best. Therefore, it is essential for general well-being and longevity to recognize the importance of cardiovascular health and take steps to maintain it.

The circulatory system is made up of capillaries, veins, arteries, and the heart. The arteries transport oxygenated blood from the heart to different regions of the body, and the veins return deoxygenated blood to the heart, acting as the central pump that circulates blood throughout the body. At the cellular level, capillaries enable the exchange of waste materials, nutrients, and oxygen. For someone to stay well and perform at their peak, the entire system needs to work in unison.

The Value of Heart and Vascular Health

1. **Preventing Cardiovascular illnesses:** The prevention of cardiovascular illnesses is one of the main justifications for placing a high priority on cardiovascular health. Poor cardiovascular health frequently leads to diseases like coronary artery disease, heart attacks, strokes, and hypertension. These illnesses can significantly lower a person's quality of life and could be fatal. A robust cardiovascular system is the first line of defense against these conditions.

2. **Prolonging Life:** Life expectancy and cardiovascular health are strongly correlated. A longer and healthier life is more likely to be supported by a cardiovascular system that is in good working order. People can lower their risk of cardiovascular illnesses and

improve their chances of leading active, meaningful lives well into old age by adopting a heart-healthy lifestyle.

3. **Improving Physical Performance:** For the best possible physical performance, a healthy cardiovascular system is essential. Good cardiovascular health makes sure that your body can effectively provide oxygen and nutrients to your muscles, enabling you to perform better and recover more quickly, whether you're an athlete or just enjoy regular physical activity.

4. **Supporting Brain Health:** Cognitive function depends on the brain receiving enough blood and oxygen. Reducing the risk of illnesses like dementia and cognitive decline, which are linked to poor blood flow to the brain, can be achieved by maintaining cardiovascular health.

5. **Increasing Energy:** Your body will get enough oxygen and nutrients if your cardiovascular system is robust, which might help you feel less tired and have more energy. This is essential for going about daily business as well as preserving a good standard of living.

6. **Managing Weight and Metabolism:** Metabolic and cardiovascular health are

intimately related. A healthy cardiovascular system can facilitate the management and maintenance of a healthy weight by assisting in the regulation of blood sugar levels and metabolism.

7. **Reducing Stress and Anxiety:** Maintaining a healthy lifestyle that promotes cardiovascular health and regular exercise can both improve mental health. It has been demonstrated that exercise improves general mental health by lowering stress and anxiety.

8. **Improving Quality of Life:** Living a cardiovascular-healthy lifestyle involves more than just preventing diseases; it also means having a higher standard of living. People who have a healthy heart and circulatory system can age independently and participate in a variety of activities.

Strategies for Enhancing Cardiovascular Health:

1. **Frequent Exercise:** One of the best strategies to support cardiovascular health is to engage in physical activity. Walking, jogging, swimming, and cycling are examples of aerobic exercises that can

strengthen the heart, promote cardiovascular fitness overall, and improve blood circulation.

2. **Balanced Diet:** Heart health can be supported by eating a diet high in fruits, vegetables, whole grains, lean protein, and healthy fats. Cutting back on sugar, salt, and saturated and trans fats can help reduce the risk of heart disease.

3. **Give Up Smoking:** One of the main risk factors for cardiovascular illnesses is smoking. One of the most effective things you can do to enhance your cardiovascular health is to give up smoking.

4. **Control Stress:** Prolonged stress can harm the heart and circulatory system. Use stress-reduction strategies like meditation, mindfulness, and relaxation techniques.

5. **Keep Your Weight in Check:** Reaching and keeping a healthy weight helps lessen the burden on your heart and minimize your chance of developing heart disease.

6. **Manage Blood Pressure:** One of the biggest risk factors for cardiovascular illnesses is high blood pressure. Maintaining and controlling your blood pressure on a regular basis can help save your heart.

7. **Control Your Cholesterol:** Excessive blood levels of LDL (bad) cholesterol can cause

plaque to accumulate in your arteries. To assist control cholesterol levels, a heart-healthy diet and, if needed, medicines are recommended.

8. **Limit Alcohol use:** The cardiovascular system may suffer from excessive alcohol use. It's imperative to either limit or stay away from alcohol completely.

9. **Get Regular Check-Ups:** Routine check-ups and screenings at a medical facility can help determine and manage cardiovascular disease risk factors.

10. **Remain Hydrated:** Sustaining blood pressure and volume requires adequate hydration. To keep your cardiovascular system healthy, make sure you are getting enough water.

cardiovascular health is essential to general wellbeing and long life. People of all ages should prioritize understanding its importance and taking proactive measures to preserve and develop it. A heart-healthy lifestyle can lower a person's risk of cardiovascular diseases and help them live longer, healthier lives with better physical and mental health. This lifestyle includes regular exercise, a balanced diet, stress management, and frequent health check-ups.

Risk Factors for Cardiovascular Disease

Undoubtedly, coronary artery disease, heart failure, stroke, and other disorders affecting the heart and blood vessels fall under the large category of cardiovascular disease (CVD). It is one of the main causes of death and disability in the world. Although heredity may contribute to an individual's susceptibility to cardiovascular disease, numerous risk variables can be altered by dietary adjustments and pharmacological therapies. We will examine the main risk factors for cardiovascular disease in this thorough discussion, including the modifiable and non-modifiable risk factors.

1. **Age:** An important, non-modifiable risk factor for cardiovascular disease is becoming older. An individual's chance of acquiring CVD rises with age. This is due to the fact that during time, the body experiences a variety of physiological changes that may aid in the development of CVD. Examples of these changes include the buildup of fatty deposits in blood vessels and the stiffening of artery walls. After the age of 65, the risk starts to significantly increase.

2. **Gender**: The risk of CVD is also influenced by gender. Compared to premenopausal women, men typically have a higher risk of CVD. But following menopause, women's risk rises and eventually catches up to men's. It is thought that the hormone estrogen, which is present in women, protects the cardiovascular system against aging-related damage.

3. **Family History:** An individual's risk may be raised if there is a history of cardiovascular disease in their family. It increases the possibility that a person may also be genetically susceptible to cardiovascular disease (CVD) if a close relative such as a parent or sibling has experienced a heart attack, stroke, or other cardiovascular problems.

4. **Genetics:** Certain genetic variables can also contribute to cardiovascular disease, even if family history is a major role. Elevated low-density lipoprotein (LDL) cholesterol is a key risk factor for cardiovascular disease (CVD) and can be caused by certain genetic disorders, such as familial hypercholesterolemia.

5. **High Blood Pressure:** One of the most important modifiable risk factors for CVD is

hypertension, or high blood pressure. Elevated blood pressure increases the risk of heart disease, stroke, and other consequences by placing additional strain on the heart and blood vessels.

6. **High Cholesterol:** A higher risk of CVD is linked to higher levels of LDL cholesterol and lower levels of HDL cholesterol. LDL cholesterol can accumulate and form plaques on the inside of artery walls, narrowing the artery and obstructing blood flow.

7. **Smoking:** One of the main risk factors for CVD is smoking. It weakens blood arteries, lowers blood oxygen levels, and promotes blood clot formation. Secondhand smoke exposure also offers a risk.

8. **Diabetes**: There is a substantial correlation between diabetes, particularly type 2 diabetes, and cardiovascular disease. Elevated blood sugar levels raise the risk of heart disease and stroke by damaging blood vessels and neurons.

9. **Obesity**: Carrying too much weight around the abdomen increases the risk of cardiovascular disease (CVD). Other risk factors like diabetes, high cholesterol, and

blood pressure are frequently connected to obesity.

10. **Physical Inactivity:** A higher risk of cardiovascular disease is linked to a lack of consistent physical activity. Exercise lowers blood pressure, strengthens the heart and lungs, and aids in maintaining a healthy weight.

11. **Unhealthy Diet:** Heart disease can arise as a result of a diet heavy in cholesterol, sodium, added sweets, saturated and trans fats, and cholesterol. On the other hand, a diet high in whole grains, fruits, vegetables, and lean meats can help reduce the risk.

12. **Excessive Alcohol Consumption:** Excessive drinking raises the risk of cardiovascular disease (CVD), high blood pressure, and other health issues, even while moderate drinking may have some cardiovascular advantages.

13. **Stress**: Extended periods of stress can result in unhealthy eating, smoking, and inactivity all of which raise the risk of CVD. Stress hormones also have the ability to raise blood pressure and induce inflammation.

14. **Sleep Apnea:** This condition, which causes breathing to stop during sleep, is linked to a

higher risk of heart disease, obesity, and hypertension.

15. **Poor Dental Health:** New studies point to a connection between cardiovascular disease and gum disease, or periodontitis. Gum disease-related inflammation may exacerbate atherosclerosis.

16. **Environmental and work Exposures:** Certain work hazards and exposure to environmental pollutants, like air pollution, can raise the risk of CVD.

17. **Inflammation illnesses:** A higher risk of cardiovascular disease has been linked to chronic inflammation illnesses such as lupus and rheumatoid arthritis.

18. **Metabolic Syndrome:** A group of illnesses that greatly raise the risk of cardiovascular disease (CVD) including high blood pressure, high blood sugar, excessive triglycerides, and abdominal obesity.

19. **Poor Medication Adherence:** The risk of CVD might be increased by failing to take prescribed drugs as indicated for diseases like diabetes or hypertension.

cardiovascular disease is a complicated illness that is impacted by a number of risk factors, both modifiable and non-modifiable. There are numerous lifestyle changes that may be made to lower the chance of having CVD, even if some factors, like age and genetics, are unchangeable. It's critical that people understand these risk factors and collaborate with medical experts to create treatment and preventative plans. A heart-healthy diet, frequent exercise, and stress reduction are just a few of the lifestyle modifications that can significantly lower the risk of cardiovascular disease.

Pritikin's Heart-Healthy Philosophy

Nathan Pritikin created the Pritikin Program in the middle of the 20th century, and it has long been acknowledged as a ground-breaking and all-encompassing strategy for leading a heart-healthy lifestyle. Pritikin's concept incorporates a comprehensive approach to general well-being, going beyond simple dietary recommendations and exercise regimens. This style of thinking has not only helped a great deal of people get better at managing their heart health, but it has also cleared the path for a more comprehensive understanding of the relationship between cardiovascular health, fitness, and nutrition.

Gaining insight from Nathan Pritikin

After receiving a heart disease diagnosis at the age of 42, Nathan Pritikin, an engineer by profession, became motivated to investigate the relationship between diet and heart health. He got into scientific research and started experimenting with food and lifestyle modifications because he was unwilling to accept a future of deteriorating health and medication. As a result of his travels, Pritikin created a program designed to both prevent and treat cardiac disease. His research raised questions about accepted medical knowledge and prompted the development of the Pritikin Program.

The Four Foundations of Pritikin's Thought

1. **Nutrition:** A diet that prioritizes whole, natural foods especially fruits, vegetables, whole grains, and legumes is the cornerstone of the Pritikin Program. A low-fat, low-cholesterol diet, according to Pritikin, may be a very effective means of avoiding and even curing heart disease. He promoted a plant-based diet that reduces the intake of processed foods, animal products,

and saturated fats. This heart-healthy diet lowers the risk of several chronic diseases, helps with weight control, and promotes cardiovascular health.

2. **Exercise**:The Pritikin philosophy places a strong emphasis on physical activity. Frequent exercise lowers the risk of heart disease, enhances cardiovascular health, and helps people maintain a healthy weight. The Pritikin program promotes strength training, flexibility training, and moderate aerobic exercise. Combining these exercises promotes general fitness and wellbeing in addition to heart health.

3. **Knowledge:** A key component of Pirtikin's philosophy is the significance of knowledge for making well-informed decisions on diet and health. Participants in the program receive the information and resources necessary to comprehend how their lifestyle and food choices affect their heart health. Meal planning, reading food labels, and comprehending the science underlying the Pritikin technique are all included in this lesson.

4. **Mind-Body Connection:** The philosophy of Pirtikin acknowledges the significant influence of stress on cardiovascular health.

He thought that in addition to bodily health, mental and emotional well-being is equally crucial. The program incorporates techniques including stress management, relaxation, and meditation to help people feel less stressed and live better overall.

Scientific Support

Pritikin's method is distinguished by its basis in scientific study. Numerous research conducted over time have attested to the Pritikin Program's efficacy in promoting heart health. Studies have indicated that individuals can improve their overall cardiovascular fitness and significantly lower their blood pressure, body weight, and cholesterol levels.

The Entire Pritikin Legacy

Long after his death, Nathan Pritikin's heart-healthy attitude continues to influence people. Numerous people have benefited from the Pritikin Program by improving their general health, preventing and treating cardiac disease, and living better lives. Additionally, Pritikin's groundbreaking research has impacted various diet and lifestyle plans and expanded knowledge of the connection between exercise, nutrition, and heart health.

The heart-healthy concept of Pritikin is a comprehensive approach to wellness that acknowledges the role that education, exercise, diet, and the mind-body link play in preserving heart health. Preventive cardiology has greatly benefited from Nathan Pritikin's devotion to research and his unshakable desire to assist people in leading better lives. His ideas still serve as a source of inspiration and direction for anyone seeking heart health and general well-being.

Crafting Your Pritikin Cardiovascular Blueprint

People all throughout the world are very concerned about their cardiovascular health. Cardiovascular illnesses continue to be the primary cause of death and morbidity, hence it is imperative to maintain a healthy heart. Thankfully, there is a tried-and-true method for enhancing heart health called the Pritikin Program. Dr. Nathan Pritikin created a comprehensive lifestyle regimen that has improved the health of thousands of people by lowering their risk of heart disease. We will explore creating your Pritikin Cardiovascular Blueprint in this post, which is a customized manual for improving your heart health.

Comprehending the Pritikin Initiative

The Pritikin Program is based on a heart-healthy lifestyle that prioritizes stress reduction, regular exercise, and a nutritious diet. Together, these pillars can lower risk factors for cardiovascular disorders like obesity, high cholesterol, and hypertension. The first step in creating your Pritikin Cardiovascular Blueprint is to have a firm grasp of these fundamental ideas.

Nutrition: The Essential Component

A diet high in whole, unprocessed foods is a fundamental component of the Pritikin Program. This strategy emphasizes eating lots of fruits, vegetables, healthy grains, and lean meats and limiting your intake of salt, added sweets, and saturated fats. A low-fat, low-sodium diet is encouraged by the program in order to lower cholesterol and keep blood pressure within normal ranges. Taking these guidelines and adapting them to your own requirements and tastes can help you create your own nutritional blueprint.

Engaging in Physical Activity: Achieving Heart Health

Frequent exercise is yet another crucial component of the Pritikin Program. Maintaining a healthy weight, enhancing cardiovascular fitness, and improving general health are all facilitated by participating in aerobic, strength, and flexibility workouts. Whether you like to walk, swim, or dance, your Pritikin Cardiovascular Blueprint should include an activity program customized to your talents and goals.

Stress Reduction: Discovering Inner Calm

Prolonged stress can raise blood pressure and cause inflammation in the body, which can lead to cardiovascular disease. The Pritikin Program places a strong emphasis on stress management methods like mindfulness, meditation, and relaxation exercises. To support heart health and emotional well-being, these stress-reduction techniques should be incorporated into your unique blueprint.

Creating a Cardiovascular Blueprint with Pritikin

Now that we have a solid understanding of the essential elements of the Pritikin Program, let's talk about how to create your unique cardiovascular blueprint:

Speak with a Medical Professional

It's crucial to speak with your healthcare practitioner before making any lifestyle changes. They can evaluate your present state of health, talk to you about any current illnesses, and offer advice on how to modify the Pritikin Program to suit your particular requirements.

Make sensible goals

The first step in creating your Pritikin Cardiovascular Blueprint is establishing specific, attainable objectives. Whether your goal is to lower your cholesterol, lose weight, or get more fit, setting clear goals will keep you motivated and on track.

Make a Customized Dietary Program

Create a specialized dietary strategy that adheres to the Pritikin principles by working with a licensed dietitian. They may assist you in figuring out how many calories you need each day, balancing your macronutrient intake, and designing a menu that works for your preferences and way of life.

Create a Workout Program

Make an exercise schedule that suits your hobbies and physical limitations. Mix up your program by including strength, flexibility, and cardio activities. As you get more fit, gradually up the intensity and length of your workouts.

Accept Stress-Reduction Strategies

Include stress-reduction strategies in your everyday activities. Try out some deep breathing techniques, mindfulness exercises, or meditation to see what works for you. These methods will safeguard your heart while assisting you in managing the difficulties of life.

Track Your Development

Maintain a log of your food decisions, exercise regimen, and stress-reduction techniques to monitor your progress on a regular basis. This will assist you in celebrating your accomplishments and identifying areas where your strategy may need to be adjusted.

Seek Assistance

Seek the assistance of loved ones, friends, or a support group that is as dedicated to heart health as you are. A network of people who share your objectives can be a great source of inspiration and support.

Creating your own Pritikin Cardiovascular Blueprint is a path to a more joyful and healthy heart. Through the adoption of the Pritikin Program's tenets, adaptation to your own circumstances, and upholding consistency, you can dramatically lower your risk of cardiovascular illnesses and lead a more satisfying life. To guarantee that you always have the best possible heart health, your blueprint is a live document that may change as you do. You may start your journey to a healthier heart and a better future with the correct direction, willpower, and assistance.

CHAPTER 4:
CHOLESTEROL REDUCTION STRATEGIES

Understanding Cholesterol

One important and frequently misinterpreted substance in the human body is cholesterol. It is an extremely important topic for health and wellness and is essential to many physiological functions. This thorough guide will cover the definition of cholesterol, its physiological roles, the various forms of cholesterol, their implications on health, and strategies for controlling cholesterol levels for optimum wellbeing.

What is cholesterol

- In every human cell, there is a waxy, fat-like material called cholesterol.
- It is necessary for several biological processes, including the synthesis of hormones, vitamin D, and cell membranes.
- It's not required to eat cholesterol; the liver may manufacture it on its own.

- On the other hand, the foods you eat can affect blood cholesterol levels.

Cholesterol and Health

- Although cholesterol is essential, an unbalanced level can cause health issues.
- Elevated "bad cholesterol" (LDL) is a significant cardiovascular disease risk factor.
- LDL cholesterol can accumulate in the walls of arteries, causing atherosclerosis and a higher risk of heart attacks and strokes.
- HDL or "good cholesterol" aids in the removal of cholesterol from arteries and returns it to the liver for excretion.
- Triglycerides are also carried by very low-density lipoprotein (VLDL), which when high can aggravate cardiac disease.

Cholesterol Testing

- Triglycerides, LDL, HDL, and total cholesterol are all measured by a lipid profile blood test.
- Knowing your lipid profile makes determining your risk of heart disease easier.

- There are guidelines that make it easier to evaluate cholesterol readings and decide if they are high or healthy.

Cholesterol Synthesis

- The majority of the cholesterol in the body is made by the liver.
- The liver can make up for dietary cholesterol intake, thus it's not as important.
- Elevated blood cholesterol levels can result from eating too much cholesterol.

Transfer of Cholesterol

- The bloodstream's carriers of lipids and cholesterol are called lipoproteins.
- LDL can build up in arterial walls and carries cholesterol from the liver to cells.
- HDL transports cholesterol back to the liver for excretion from cells and arteries.
- Triglycerides are a kind of fat that are carried by VLDL, which can also aggravate heart disease.

Managing Cholesterol

- Modifying one's lifestyle is crucial for lowering cholesterol.
- Lowering LDL cholesterol and raising HDL cholesterol helps lessen the risk of heart disease, as does quitting smoking, exercising frequently, and maintaining a balanced diet.
- When dietary modifications alone aren't sufficient to lower cholesterol, doctors may recommend medications like fibrates and statins.
- Reducing saturated and trans fats, upping fiber consumption, and selecting foods that can lower cholesterol are all part of a heart-healthy diet.

MYTHS AND FACTS ABOUT CHOLESTEROL

- **Myth:** There is no good cholesterol.
- **Fact:** The right amount of cholesterol depends on the balance of the various forms.

- **Myth:** Eating meals high in cholesterol always causes blood cholesterol levels to rise.
- **Fact:** For most people, dietary cholesterol has no effect on blood cholesterol levels.
- **Myth:** All fats raise cholesterol levels.
- Unsaturated fats are good for the heart; not all fats are bad.
- **Myth:** The only way to manage cholesterol is through medication.
- **Fact:** Changing one's diet and exercising helps control cholesterol levels quite a little.

Maintaining good health and preventing significant medical disorders require an understanding of cholesterol. People can take charge of their cholesterol levels and lower their risk of heart disease and other health issues by understanding the function of various forms of cholesterol, interpreting the findings of cholesterol tests, and adopting educated dietary and lifestyle decisions. It all comes down to fostering wellbeing and striking a healthy balance.

Pritikin's Approach to Cholesterol Management

Nathan Pritikin created the Pritikin Program in the 1950s, which is a comprehensive lifestyle program for controlling cholesterol and enhancing cardiovascular health in general. It stresses a trifecta of dietary adjustments, consistent exercise, and stress reduction. The Pritikin approach to cholesterol management, which has been helpful in lowering people's cholesterol levels and heart disease risk, is examined in this article along with its main ideas and constituent parts.

Pritikin Diet

Prioritizing Low Fat and High Fiber

Whole, unprocessed foods including fruits, vegetables, whole grains, legumes, and lean protein sources that are naturally high in fiber and low in fat are the foundation of the Pritikin diet.

A key component of this strategy is lowering dietary fat intake, especially saturated and trans fats, which can raise LDL cholesterol levels.

Reducing Consumption of Cholesterol

1. Pritikin advocates for a diet that is almost devoid of foods high in cholesterol, like red meat, whole-fat dairy products, and egg yolks.
2. It highlights the use of foods like beans, soy products, and oats that decrease cholesterol.

Control of Portion

1. Portion control is encouraged by the program to aid with weight management because carrying extra weight might raise cholesterol levels.
2. Reducing calories and portion sizes are two important tactics for keeping a healthy weight.

Consistent Exercise:

Exercises Aerobic:

Pritikin suggests doing aerobic exercises like cycling, swimming, or brisk walking on a daily basis.

Lowering LDL cholesterol and increasing HDL cholesterol the "good" cholesterol are two benefits of aerobic exercise.

Exercises for Strength

1. Strength training activities contribute to the development of lean muscle mass, which enhances cardiovascular health and metabolism.
2. It is a crucial component of the Pritikin program's general fitness component.

Changes in Lifestyle

Stress Reduction

1. Stress can be a factor in both unhealthy eating patterns and high cholesterol.

2. In order to support emotional wellbeing, Pritikin promotes stress-reduction methods like mindfulness, relaxation training, and meditation.

Giving Up Smoking

1. Smoking can have a detrimental effect on cholesterol levels and is a major risk factor for heart disease.
2. The Pritikin program offers assistance and resources to those who want to give up smoking.

Research and Scientific Foundations

The Pritikin Center for Longevity:

1. Nathan Pritikin developed the Pritikin Longevity Center and Spa, which provides complete lifestyle education and cholesterol management through residential programs.
2. These programs are the result of many years of clinical and research experience.

Studies on the Efficacy of Pritikin:

1. The Pritikin program can significantly lower LDL cholesterol and overall cardiovascular risk, according to a number of studies.
2. Studies validate the efficaciousness of a diet rich in fiber and low in fat when paired with consistent exercise to enhance cholesterol levels and foster cardiovascular well-being.

Obstacles and Things to Think About:

Modifications to Diet:

1. Those used to a diet heavy in processed foods and saturated fats may find it difficult to adjust to the Pritikin diet.
2. It calls for both dedication and a readiness to alter one's diet significantly.

Consistent Use Over Time:

1. Some people may find it challenging to stick with the Pritikin program over the long run since it requires significant lifestyle changes.

2. Success can sometimes depend on continued assistance and education.

The Pritikin method of cholesterol control provides a comprehensive lifestyle plan that incorporates regular exercise, stress reduction, a high-fiber, low-fat diet, and other healthful practices. It has been demonstrated that its emphasis on natural, whole foods and low dietary fat has a beneficial effect on cholesterol levels and general cardiovascular health. The research demonstrates its effectiveness in lowering the risk of heart disease and encouraging a healthy, cholesterol-friendly lifestyle, even if it may necessitate a major commitment.

CHAPTER 5: THE PRITIKIN PLATE: A BLUEPRINT FOR HEALTH

Mastering the Pritikin Plate

Eating a balanced diet may be made easy and effective with the Pritikin Plate. It has been demonstrated to be beneficial in preventing and treating heart disease, stroke, and other chronic illnesses. It is founded on the ideas of eating a diet high in complex carbohydrates and low in fat.

There are three portions on the Pritikin Plate:

- **Whole grains and complex carbohydrates:** Whole-wheat bread and pasta, brown rice, quinoa, oats, and starchy vegetables like potatoes, corn, and peas are good sources of whole grains and complex carbs.

- **Fruits and vegetables:** Reserve another quarter of your plate for this category. Aim for a rainbow of hues in your fruits and vegetables, including melons, berries, citrus fruits, and leafy greens.

- **Lean protein:** The last part of your plate should consist of this area. Tofu, fish, chicken, beans, lentils, and fowl are good sources of lean protein.

The Pritikin Plate also highlights the significance of reducing added sugar, cholesterol, and saturated and trans fats. Your risk of heart disease, stroke, and other chronic illnesses may increase if you consume certain nutrients.

Here are some tips for mastering the Pritikin Plate:

1. **Choose whole grains over refined grains:** Fibre, vitamins, and minerals can be found in abundance in whole grains. Conversely, refined grains have less nutritious value because the bran and germ have been removed.

2. **Consume a lot of fruits and veggies:** Vegetables and fruits are abundant in vitamins, minerals, and antioxidants but low in calories. Consume five servings or more of fruits and vegetables each day.

3. **Choose lean protein sources:** Low in cholesterol and saturated fat are sources of lean protein. Tofu, fish, chicken, beans, lentils, and fowl are good sources of lean protein.

4. **Limit saturated and trans fats:** You run a higher risk of heart disease and higher cholesterol when you consume trans and saturated fats. Choose lean protein sources, stay away from processed foods, and use healthy cooking oils like canola and olive oil to reduce your intake of saturated and trans fats.

5. **Limit cholesterol:** Your risk of heart disease can rise along with your cholesterol levels when you consume cholesterol. Choose lean protein sources and stay away from items high in cholesterol, like organ meats, egg yolks, and full-fat dairy products, to reduce your intake of cholesterol.

6. **Limit sugar additions:** Sugar additions may be a factor in weight gain and other medical issues. Restrict your consumption of added sugar by staying away from processed meals, sweets, and sugary drinks.

An example of a day's food plan using the Pritikin Plate is as follows:

BREAKFAST

- Nuts and berries in oatmeal
- Avocado and tomato on whole-wheat bread
- granola and fruit paired with yogurt

LUNCHTIME

- salad topped with fish or barbecued chicken
- Lentil soup
- Place hummus, veggies, and lean protein on a whole-wheat sandwich.

DINNER

- Roasted veggie and salmon
- Quinoa salad with corn and black beans
- Stir-fried chicken over brown rice

SNACKS:

- Fruits and vegetables
- Nuts and seeds
- Yogurt

You may enhance your health, lower your chance of developing chronic diseases, and lose weight by following the Pritikin Plate, which is a nutritious and well-balanced diet. You may master the Pritikin Plate and reap all of its benefits by paying attention to the advice provided above.

Here are some more pointers for being proficient with the Pritikin Plate:

Plan your meals ahead of time: This will assist you in avoiding unhealthy snacking and making wise decisions.

Make as much food as you can at home: In this manner, you can keep an eye on the components in your food and steer clear of harmful chemicals.

Make healthy substitutions: For instance, use avocado or olive oil in place of butter. Use quinoa or brown rice in place of white rice.

Don't be afraid to experiment: The Pritikin Plate rules can be followed to create a variety of tasty and healthful foods.

Pritikin Plate is a lifestyle shift. Gaining mastery of it requires time and work. However, the Pritikin Plate can help you live a longer, healthier life and enhance your health, therefore it is worth it.

Food Groups and Servings

Being aware of food types and serving sizes is essential to eating a healthy diet. It's important to consider both what you eat and how much of each food type you take in. This information enables people to make wise decisions, guaranteeing a healthy diet that is balanced and nutritious. We will examine the various food groups and suggested portion sizes in this investigation, assisting you in making better decisions every day.

The Required Dietary Groups

Foods fall into several basic categories, which are crucial to understand in order to understand food groupings and portions. These dietary groups fulfill specific roles in the body's operation and offer a variety of vital nutrients.

The key food groups include:

1. **Fruits**: Packed full of fiber, natural sugars, vitamins, and minerals are fruits. From citrus fruits like oranges to berries and tropical fruits like pineapples, they are available in a wide range of varieties. Eating a wide variety of fruits offers a wide range of nutrients.

2. **Vegetables**: Packed with vitamins, minerals, and dietary fiber, vegetables are nutritional powerhouses. This group includes leafy greens, cruciferous veggies like broccoli, and colorful alternatives like carrots.

3. **Grains**: Whole grains are best since they contain more of their natural nutrients and fiber, like whole wheat, quinoa, and oats.

4. **Protein**: Sources from both plants and animals are included in the protein group. Meat, poultry, and fish are examples of animal sources; beans,

lentils, tofu, and nuts are examples of plant-based sources. Among its many crucial uses, protein is necessary for the healing of muscles and tissues.

5. **Dairy (or Alternatives):** Calcium and vitamin D are abundant in dairy products including milk, yogurt, and cheese. For those who have a lactose intolerance or would rather consume plant-based foods, fortified nut cheeses, soy yogurt, and almond milk are good substitutes.

6. **Fats**: Although they aren't usually thought of as their own food group, fats are an important part of the diet. Nuts, olive oil, avocados, and other foods are good sources of healthy fats. They promote a number of body processes and offer vital fatty acids.

Recommended Servings

It's crucial to balance these food groups in your diet on a regular basis to make sure you're getting a variety of nutrients. Your needs for servings vary depending on your age, sex, exercise level, and general health objectives. But here are some broad pointers to get you going:

- **Fruits and Vegetables:** Try to have half of your plate composed of these items. This entails eating at least five servings of fruits and vegetables each day for the majority of individuals.

- **Grain**: Whenever feasible, opt for whole grains. Six to eight servings of grains a day, primarily whole grains, should be the goal for adults.

- **Protein**: Make sure your diet includes a range of protein sources. Adults require 5 to 7 ounces of protein on average per day, which should include a combination of lean meat, chicken, fish, and plant-based foods.

- **Dairy:** To achieve their daily requirements for calcium and vitamin D, adults usually need three servings of dairy or dairy replacements.

- **Fats**: Limiting saturated and trans fats and consuming healthy fats in moderation are important, even though there is no set daily serving requirement for fats.

- **Sweets and treats**: These have minimal nutritional value and frequently contain excess calories, therefore they should be consumed in moderation.

Practical Tips for Balanced Nutrition

Take into account these helpful suggestions to maintain a balanced diet with the appropriate food groups and serving sizes:

- **Meal Planning:** Make sure each food group is fairly represented in your meal plans. As a result, no category is over consumed.

- **Read Labels:** Read food labels carefully to learn about portion sizes and the nutritional makeup of packaged goods.

- **Portion Control:** To precisely portion your food and avoid overindulging, use scales and measuring glasses.

- **Cook at Home:** You can have more control over the ingredients and portion proportions when you prepare your meals at home.

- **Speak with a Dietitian:** A licensed dietitian can offer tailored advice if you have certain dietary requirements or health objectives.

A healthy lifestyle is built on a foundation of balanced eating. You may make decisions that improve your general quality of life and promote your well-being by being aware of dietary groups and suggested serving sizes.

Meal Planning Made Simple

Meal planning is a potent tool that may change the way you feel about food, help you save time and money, and improve your general health and wellbeing. Acquiring the skill of meal planning can simplify your life and improve the quality of your meals, regardless of your experience level in household cooking. We'll walk you through the meal planning process in this article, providing you with easy-to-follow advice and techniques to get you started and help you stick to a regular meal planning schedule.

The Significance of Meal Planning

Making a grocery list and selecting what to eat for supper are only two aspects of meal planning. It's a thorough strategy that includes planning ahead, choosing your food wisely, and coordinating your meals with your overall lifestyle and health objectives. Meal planning is crucial for the following reasons:

Saves Time: Arranging your meals in advance can help you to free up valuable time throughout the workweek. There won't be any more hurried trips to the grocery store or last-minute meal planning after a demanding day.

Saves Money: You may lower your grocery costs by making thoughtful ingredient purchases and minimizing food waste.

Health Benefits: You may manage your weight, heart health, and general well-being by meal planning, which enables you to make wholesome decisions and regulate portion sizes.

Variety and Creativity: Organizing your meals allows you to experiment with new dishes, ingredients, and cooking methods, which will delight you as you go on your culinary adventure.

Decreased Stress: Planning your meals for the week helps you eat more comfortably by easing the tension and worry that comes with mealtimes.

Easy Steps to Plan Your Meals

Make a Goal List: Determine your goals for meal planning first. Do you want to cut down on food waste, save time, or adopt a better diet? Your process of meal planning will be guided by your goals.

Make a Weekly Menu: Arrange your meals, including breakfast, lunch, dinner, and snacks, for the coming week. Make a list of your options in a plain notebook or a calendar.

Pick meals: Make sure the meals you choose fit your dietary restrictions and objectives. For ideas, look through recipe books, food blogs, or meal planning apps and websites.

Examine Your Pantry: Determine what is currently in your freezer, refrigerator, and pantry. By doing this, you can cut down on waste and prevent purchasing duplicate ingredients.

Make a Shopping List: Make a thorough shopping list based on the recipes you've selected and the items you'll need. For a more efficient grocery trip, arrange it according to food categories.

Prepare Ahead: Complete some prep work ahead of time to save time throughout the workweek. This could involve preparing grains ahead of time, marinating meats, or chopping veggies.

Be Adaptable: Although preparation is necessary, it's critical to maintain flexibility. As life can bring you unforeseen twists and turns, adjust your plan accordingly.

Portion Control: Take into account serving sizes and don't put too much food on one plate. This will lessen food waste and assist you in controlling your calorie consumption.

Variety Is Important: To make sure you obtain a wide range of nutrients, try to eat a variety of meals, such as different grains, fruits, vegetables, and meats.

Track Your Development: Evaluate the success of your food planning after a week. What was effective and what could be made better? Make use of this input to improve your strategy.

Tools for Meal Planning

A plethora of tools exist to further streamline meal planning:

Meal Planning applications: You may find recipes that fit your dietary requirements, make shopping lists, and plan your meals with the aid of a variety of smartphone applications.

Cookbooks: Get a few high-quality cookbooks that complement your culinary hobbies and aspirations. They can be quite helpful as inspiration sources.

Online Recipe Databases: There are a ton of recipe websites and blogs on the internet that provide a ton of food ideas.

Meal Planning Templates: To assist you in organizing your weekly menu and shopping list, you can find printable meal planning templates online.

Meal planning is a simple yet powerful habit that can improve your eating patterns, simplify your daily schedule, and lead to a happier, healthier life. You can master meal planning and enjoy all of its advantages by following the instructions in this guide and using useful tools. So go ahead and prepare your meals now, and enjoy the convenience and fulfillment they offer to your kitchen.

CHAPTER 6: THE 2024 PRITIKIN DIET PLAN

A Week of Sample Menus

A great method to make sure you're fulfilling your nutritional needs and tasting a range of flavors and ingredients is to plan a week's worth of balanced meals. Here, we offer a sample week's worth of dinners that accommodate various dietary requirements and objectives. Whether your goal is to enhance your health, manage your weight, or just broaden your culinary horizons, these meals are meant to serve as inspiration and a tool for creating your own meal plans.

Day 1: Mediterranean Delight

Breakfast

- Greek yogurt paired with a blend of berries and honey
- Whole-grain bread for lunch

Lunch

- Mediterranean salad with feta cheese, tomatoes, cucumbers, and olives
- Whole-grain pita bread and hummus

Dinner

- Chicken grilled with oregano and lemon
- Quinoa paired with roasted veggies
- Sauce Tzatziki

Snack

- Dates and dehydrated apricots

Day 2: Paradise Plant-Based

Breakfast

- Toast with avocado and cherry tomatoes
- Fresh fruit salad

Lunch

- Curry with lentils and vegetables
- Brown rice

Dinner

- Bell peppers filled with black beans and quinoa
- Steaming broccoli

Snack

- Cucumber and carrot sticks with hummus

Day 3: Protein Packed

Breakfast

- Feta cheese and spinach added to scrambled eggs
- Whole-grain bread

Lunch

- Wrap with avocado and turkey and whole-wheat tortilla
- salad of mixed greens with balsamic dressing

Dinner

- Fish baked with herbs and lemon
- Steamed asparagus with quinoa as a

Snack

- Greek yogurt topped with honeydew and sliced bananas

Day 4: Comfort Classics

Breakfast

- Banana slices and cinnamon sprinkled over oatmeal
- Low-fat milk or a substitute for milk

Lunchtime

- Sandwich made with grilled cheese and whole-grain bread
- Tomato soup

Dinner

- Turkey meatballs and marinara sauce on spaghetti
- Steaming broccoli

Snack

- Slices of apple with peanut butter

Day 5: International Flavors

Breakfast

- Spanish omelette with onions and bell peppers
- Orange slices

Lunch

- Pho Vietnamese with tofu and an abundance of herbs
- Served with peanut dipping sauce, fresh spring rolls

Dinner

- Butter chicken prepared in the Indian way
- basmati rice
- naan bread;

Snack

- Mango lassi
- Smoothie made with yogurt.

Day 6: A Fast and Healthful

Breakfast

- Berries and whole-grain cereal
- Low-fat milk or a substitute for milk

Lunch

- Mixed veggie quinoa salad with a lemon-tahini dressing

Dinner

- Shrimp stir-fried with a variety of veggies
- Brown rice

Snack

- Cherry tomatoes and cucumber slices with a touch of balsamic vinegar

Day 7:Grill it up

Breakfast

- Spinach, banana, and protein powder smoothie
- Whole-grain bread

Launch

- Quinoa salad with grilled vegetables

Dinner

- Coleslaw and BBQ chicken
- Baked sweet potatoes

Snack

Dehydrated cranberries and mixed nuts

You can use these sample meals as a jumping off point for your own creative meal planning endeavors. Depending on your unique dietary requirements and tastes, you can change the components and quantities. To make your meals tasty and nourishing, always strive for variety, select whole, minimally processed foods, and concentrate on balanced nutrition.

Grocery Shopping the Pritikin Way

When grocery shopping is done in a Pritikin manner, it becomes a thoughtful and health-conscious activity. The Pritikin program, which is based on the ideas of Dr. Nathan Pritikin, stresses a plant-based, low-fat diet for improving general health. This is a theory that applies to the way you choose, buy, and prepare food. Here, we'll walk you through the fundamentals of grocery shopping the Pritikin way, empowering you to make wise decisions that support vitality and wellness.

The Philosophy of Pritikin

The core tenet of the Pritikin philosophy is that our health is directly influenced by the foods we eat. Dr. Nathan Pritikin thought that the secret to preventing and even curing chronic diseases was to follow a diet high in whole, natural foods, especially those that come from plants. This mindset is supported by the Pritikin method of grocery shopping, which places an emphasis on foods high in fiber and vital nutrients and low in fat.

Advice for Purchasing Grocery the Pritikin Way

Create a List Prior to shopping for groceries, make a thorough shopping list. This keeps you from making rash, unhealthy purchases while also assisting you in staying on course.

1. **Shop the Periphery:** In most supermarkets, the fresh and minimally processed produce, whole grains, lean meats, and fruits are located in the outermost sections. Shop primarily in these locations.

2. **Select Fruits and veggies:** A vibrant assortment of fruits and veggies should make up the majority of your cart. To make sure you get a wide range of important vitamins and minerals, choose a variety.

3. **Whole Grains:** Choose whole grains rather than refined ones, such as oats, brown rice, quinoa, and whole wheat pasta. They are nutritious and fiber-rich.

4. **Lean Proteins:** Select lean animal products such as fish, skinless chicken, and low-fat dairy. It is advised, nevertheless, to include plant-based proteins such tofu, lentils, and beans.

5. **Reduce Added Fats:** Look for items with little to no added oil and check labels for added fats. Unhealthy fats are frequently found in processed foods, sauces, and cooking oils.

6. **Read Labels:** Become acquainted with the labels on food items. Seek products with minimal ingredient lists and steer clear of those with a lot of added sugar, preservatives, and additives.

7. **Eat Fewer Processed meals:** Prepackaged and processed meals can include high levels of sugar, salt, and harmful fats. Reduce the number of these products in your cart.

8. **Stock Up on Herbs and Spices:** Instead of using salt or heavy sauces to enhance flavor, use herbs and spices. This enhances flavor and may provide health benefits as well.

9. **Remain Hydrated:** Remember to stay hydrated! A cart should always have an ample supply of water, herbal teas, and other low-calorie, unsweetened beverages because water is an essential component of the Pritikin lifestyle.

10. **Be Aware of Portion Sizes:** Pay attention to portion sizes even while selecting healthful foods. Your ambitions may be harmed by overindulging.

11. **Think About Organic Options:** Look into organic items if at all possible, especially for the "Dirty Dozen," which are fruits and vegetables that are more likely to have pesticide residues.

Beyond the Pritikin Lifestyle of Shopping

Embracing the Pritikin lifestyle involves more than just grocery shopping. Keep in mind that your decisions in the kitchen, how you prepare your meals, and your general attitude toward health, which includes regular exercise, are all essential elements. To make sure you're headed in the right direction toward health and wellness, ask Pritikin programs or medical professionals for advice and assistance.

Grocery shopping the Pritikin way is an intentional, health-conscious activity that supports the idea of full, plant-based eating. You may make wise decisions and incorporate the advantages of the Pritikin lifestyle into your kitchen and, eventually, your life according to the guidelines provided here.

Preparing Delicious Pritikin Meals

Making delectable Pritikin dishes is gratifying and simple. You can make tasty and healthful meals with a little preparation and imagination.

The following advice can help you make delectable Pritikin meals:

Utilize complete, fresh ingredients: The healthiest and tastiest ingredients are whole and fresh. Select locally grown and organic produce whenever feasible.
Select sources of lean protein: Tofu, fish, chicken, beans, lentils, and fowl are good sources of lean protein.
Use good fats when cooking: Nutritious fats like avocado, canola, and olive oils can enhance the taste and texture of your food.

Employ spices and herbs: Spices and herbs can improve the flavor of your food without adding bad components like fat, sugar, or salt.

Make your recipes unique: There are a ton of delectable and healthful Pritikin recipes in cookbooks and on the internet. Try out a variety of recipes to see which ones your family likes.

The following are some particular pointers for cooking delectable Pritikin meals in many categories:

Breakfast

- **Oatmeal**: An adaptable and wholesome breakfast option is oatmeal. Add spices, nuts, seeds, and berries to increase the flavor.
- **Yogurt**: Another delectable and nutritious breakfast option is yogurt. Add nuts, granola, and fruit on top.
- **Eggs**: Rich in protein and other nutrients, eggs are a great food. Serve them on whole-wheat bread or sauté them with vegetables in a scramble.

Lunch

- **Salads**: Getting your recommended daily intake of fruits and vegetables is made easy with salads. Toss in a mix of greens and veggies, and add lean protein (grilled chicken or fish, beans, lentils) to top your salad.
- **Soups**: Another filling and healthful lunch choice is soup. Serve veggie or chicken noodle soups with whole-wheat crackers or toast.
- **Sandwiches**: Put lean protein, veggies, and hummus or mustard on whole-wheat bread. Steer clear of processed cheese and meats.

Dinner

- **Fish**: Fish is a good source of omega-3 fatty acids and protein. Salmon can be baked with herbs and lemon or roasted with veggies.
- **Chicken**: Another wholesome and adaptable source of protein is chicken. Bake, grill, or stir-fry it with veggies.
- **Beans**: Rich in fiber and protein, beans are a great food choice. Use beans to make tacos, chili, or bean soup.

Snack

- **Fruits and vegetables:** These make wholesome and practical snacks. Consume them dried, frozen, or fresh.
- **Nuts and seeds:** Rich in protein and heart-healthy lipids, nuts and seeds are a great food. Consume them on their own or mix them with salads, oats, and yogurt.
- **Yogurt:** A nutritious and filling snack is yogurt. Add nuts, granola, and fruit on top.

Tasty and nutritious Pritikin meals are simple to make with a little preparation and imagination. Try out a variety of recipes and ingredients to see which ones your family likes.

Adapting the Pritikin Diet to Your Lifestyle

Low in cholesterol, added sugar, and saturated and trans fats, the Pritikin diet is a nutritious way of eating. It has a lot of fiber and complex carbs as well. Research has demonstrated the efficacy of the Pritikin diet in the prevention and treatment of heart disease, stroke, and other chronic illnesses.

Still, some people find it difficult to stick to the Pritikin diet, particularly those who lead hectic lives. The following advice can help you modify the Pritikin diet to fit your needs:

- **Arrange your snacks and meals ahead of time:** This will assist you in avoiding unwise decisions while you're pressed for time.
- **Make a lot of food on the weekends:** In this manner, you'll start the week with wholesome meals and snacks prepared.
- **Use leftovers**: Using leftovers is a terrific method to cut costs and save time. You may reheat them for dinner or pack them up for lunch.
- **Have wholesome snacks available:** This will assist you in avoiding bad snacks when you're famished. Yogurt, almonds, seeds, fruits, and veggies make healthful snack options.
- **Make healthy substitutions:** Make healthy replacements in your recipes whenever you can. For instance, use avocado or olive oil in place of butter. Use quinoa or brown rice in place of white rice.

The following particular advice can be used to modify the Pritikin diet to fit various lifestyles:

Busy professionals

- **The night before, make your lunch and breakfast plans**: You'll be able to avoid making harmful decisions and save time in the morning by doing this.
- **Bring your own lunch and snacks:** You may choose healthy selections and maintain control over the ingredients in your diet in this way.
- **When dining out, pick nutritious selections:** Seek out eateries that serve a lot of fruits and vegetables in their baked or grilled dishes.

Pick nutritious options like fruits, veggies, nuts, seeds, and yogurt if you must eat on the run.

Families

- **Involve the entire family in the planning and preparation of meals:** Everyone's likelihood of enjoying and finishing the meals will increase as a result.
- **Pick dishes that are simple to prepare and will appeal to all palates:** There are a ton of delectable and healthful Pritikin recipes in cookbooks and on the internet.
- **Regarding your meal plan, be adaptable.** Do not hesitate to adjust your meal plan if your family has a hectic schedule. For instance, you

might have to prepare a simpler dinner or eat leftovers more frequently.

People with dietary restrictions

- **Consult a qualified nutritionist or your doctor if you have any dietary restrictions:** They can assist you in customizing the Pritikin diet to fit your unique requirements.
- **Numerous online and cookbook resources are available to help modify the Pritikin diet to accommodate various dietary constraints:** Cookbooks, for instance, are available for those who are gluten intolerant, have food allergies, or have diabetes.

A little preparation and work will allow you to simply modify the Pritikin diet to fit your needs. The Pritikin diet can help you get healthier and lower your chance of developing chronic diseases. It is a sustainable and healthful eating plan.

CHAPTER 7: PRITIKIN RECIPES FOR WELLNESS

Breakfast Masterpieces

The most significant meal of the day is breakfast, which is also a fantastic opportunity to experiment with food. Here are some mouthwatering and nutrient-dense breakfast masterpieces:

1. Avocado Toast

There's a reason avocado toast is a staple breakfast option. Not only is it really easy to prepare, but it's also quite tasty and nourishing. Avocados are an excellent source of vitamins, fiber, and beneficial fats. Simply mash one avocado and spread it over a slice of whole-wheat toast to make avocado toast. Avocado toast can be topped with a lot of different things, such tomatoes, eggs, sprouts, or a dash of chilli flakes.

2. Oatmeal with Berries and Nuts

Another adaptable and healthful breakfast choice is oatmeal. It's a fantastic source of fiber, protein, and complex carbs. Just follow the instructions on the package to prepare oatmeal and add nuts and fruit. Add some nuts and fresh berries, and if you'd like, sprinkle in some honey or maple syrup.

3. Yogurt with Fruit and Granola

A nutritious breakfast that is high in calcium and protein is yogurt. Just arrange yogurt, fruit, and granola in a bowl or jar to make yogurt with fruit and granola. Any kind of fruit will work, including apples, bananas, and berries.

4. Eggs with Vegetables

A wonderful source of protein and other nutrients is an egg. Just scramble or cook eggs with your favorite veggies, such as tomatoes, peppers, or onions, to make eggs with vegetables. Additionally, you can use vegetables to make an omelet or frittata.

5. Smoothies

A quick and simple way to have a nutritious breakfast on the run is with a smoothie. Just blend your favorite fruits, veggies, and yogurt to create a smoothie. If you want a more substantial and nourishing meal, you may also add milk or protein powder to your smoothie.

These are but a handful of inventive breakfast recipes. Find meals that you and your family will love by becoming creative and experimenting with different components.

Lunchtime Delights

Lunch is a fantastic opportunity to consume a tasty and nourishing meal. These are some delicious and healthful lunchtime options:

1. Lentil Soup

A filling, tasty soup that's high in fiber and protein is lentil soup. It is a good provider of various nutrients, including iron. Just cook lentils in broth with your preferred vegetables to make lentil soup. To taste, you can also add herbs and spices.

2. Quinoa Salad with Black Beans and Corn

A light and cool salad that's ideal for a summer lunch is quinoa salad. It is a good source of fiber, complex carbs, and protein. Just cook the quinoa per the instructions on the package to make quinoa salad. Add your preferred dressing, corn, veggies, and black beans and stir.

3. Tuna Salad Sandwich

A tuna salad sandwich is a traditional favorite for lunch. It is an excellent source of omega-3 fatty acids and protein. Simply combine tuna, mayonnaise, celery, onion, and your preferred seasonings to make a tuna salad sandwich. Enjoy the tuna salad by spreading it over two slices of whole-wheat bread.

4. Leftover Salmon with Roasted Vegetables

A simple and quick lunch option is leftover salmon with roasted veggies. It is an excellent source of omega-3 fatty acids and protein. To reheat leftover salmon and roasted veggies, just pop them back into the oven or microwave.

5. Chicken and Avocado Wrap

A filling and nutritious lunch option is a wrap with chicken and avocado. It is a wonderful source of fiber, healthy fats, and protein. Spread some hummus on a whole-wheat tortilla to assemble a chicken and avocado wrap. Add your preferred vegetables, avocado, and grilled chicken to the hummus. Sew up the tortilla and savor it.

These are just a few suggestions for delicious lunchtime fare. Find meals that you and your family will love by becoming creative and experimenting with different components.

Dinner Creations

1. Grilled Salmon with Roasted Vegetables

This is a traditional, healthful dinner choice. Roasted veggies are a wonderful amount of vitamins, minerals, and fiber; salmon is a good supply of protein and omega-3 fatty acids. Simply roast your preferred veggies in the oven and grill the salmon fillets until they are cooked through. For a full meal, serve with quinoa or brown rice on the side.

2. Chicken Stir-Fry with Brown Rice

A simple and quick dinner for a weeknight is this stir-fry. It's also a rich source of vegetables, complex carbs, and protein. Just toss chicken with your preferred veggies in a big skillet or wok. For a full meal, serve with quinoa or brown rice.

3. Pasta with Lentil Sauce

This pasta recipe is an excellent vegetarian substitute because it is high in protein and fiber. Lentils are a great source of protein, iron, and other nutrients. To cook the lentils and combine the tomatoes, garlic, and herbs to make a sauce, simply follow the directions on the package. Serve with your favorite spaghetti and grated Parmesan cheese.

4. Quinoa Bowl with Roasted Vegetables and Chickpeas

A nutritious and filling dish that's ideal for a midweek dinner is this quinoa bowl. Roasted veggies and chickpeas are wonderful sources of vitamins, minerals, and fiber; quinoa is a good source of protein, complex carbohydrates, and fiber. Just toss your favorite veggies and chickpeas into the oven to roast. Next, put the chickpeas and roasted veggies in a bowl with the quinoa and your preferred dressing. Accompany with hummus or yogurt on the side.

5. Black Bean Burgers with Sweet Potato Fries

A tasty and nutritious substitute for beef burgers are these black bean burgers. Sweet potato fries are a wonderful source of vitamins, minerals, and complex carbs; black beans are a good source of protein and fiber. To prepare the burgers, simply combine the black beans, oats, and spices. Next, cook the burgers on the grill or in the oven. Accompany with your preferred toppings and sweet potato fries.

CHAPTER 8: MONITORING YOUR PROGRESS

Tracking Your Health Metrics

Monitoring your health indicators over time will help you spot any areas where you might need to make adjustments and track your progress. You may monitor a wide range of different health parameters, such as:

- Weight
- Body mass index (BMI)
- Body fat percentage
- Blood pressure
- Heart rate
- Cholesterol levels
- Blood sugar levels
- Sleep quality
- Activity levels

You have two options for monitoring your health metrics: manually or with a range of tools like these:

- Fitness trackers
- Smartwatches
- Blood pressure monitors

- Blood glucose meters
- Sleep trackers
- Activity trackers

Once you begin monitoring your health measurements, you may utilize the information to spot patterns and trends. You can use this information to track your progress over time, create objectives, and make lifestyle improvements.

The following advice can help you monitor your health metrics:

- **Select the metrics that hold the highest significance for you.** Health measurements are not all made equal. For general health, some metrics like weight and BMI are more significant than others. Select the parameters that are most pertinent to your personal health objectives.
- **Keep a regular eye on your stats**. Monitoring your metrics on a frequent basis is essential to identifying trends and patterns. Track your measurements once a week or more frequently if you are aiming to reach a particular health objective.
- **Remain dependable.** Maintaining consistency in your tracking is essential for

reliable reporting. Try to track your metrics every day at the same time and in the same environment.

- **Apply a tracking device.** Both digital and manual tracking tools come in a multitude of varieties. Select a tracking device that will assist you in staying on course and is simple to use.
- **Regularly assess your progress.** Every week or month, set aside some time to assess your development. This will assist you in maintaining your motivation and pinpointing any areas that could require adjustment.

Monitoring your health metrics is a wonderful method to keep an eye on your health and spot any issues before they become serious. You may make well-informed decisions on your lifestyle and health by routinely monitoring your measurements and evaluating your progress over time.

Regular Check-Ins and Adjustments

Sustaining optimal health and well-being requires regular check-ins and changes. They enable you to recognize possible issues early on, deal with them, and alter your lifestyle or treatment plan as needed.

Why are routine evaluations and modifications crucial?

Adjustments and check-ins on a regular basis are crucial for several reasons. They first enable you to see possible issues early on and take appropriate action. For long-term illnesses like diabetes, heart disease, and high blood pressure, this is particularly crucial. Long-term results can be enhanced and problems can be avoided with early detection and treatment.

Second, you can modify your treatment plan or lifestyle as needed with the help of routine check-ins and adjustments. For instance, your doctor might advise modifying your diet, exercise regimen, or medication if you are not seeing results in your weight loss or blood pressure control.

Finally, you may maintain your motivation and accountability by making regular check-ins and modifications. Maintaining your health objectives can be made easier if you are aware that you have scheduled regular visits with your physician or other healthcare practitioner.

How frequently should you make routine adjustments and check-ins?

The regularity of your check-ins and adjustments will be customized for your specific health needs. You might need to visit your doctor more frequently than someone who is normally well if you have a chronic illness.

The following are general recommendations on the frequency of routine examinations and adjustments:

- **Adults**: If an adult has a chronic illness or is at high risk for a particular disease, they should get a physical examination at least once every three years.
- **Children and teenagers:** Considering their age and developmental stage, children and teenagers should see their physician or another healthcare professional on a frequent basis.
- **Pregnant Women:** Expectant mothers should visit their doctor frequently for prenatal care throughout their pregnancies.

What takes place when you do a routine check-in and adjustment?

Your physician or another healthcare professional will usually carry out the following procedures during a routine check-in and adjustment:

- **Examine your medical background.** This covers any previous operations, allergies, prescription drugs, and medical issues.
- **Do a physical examination.** This entails taking your height, weight, and vital signs. In addition, your physician might palpate your belly and listen to your heart and lungs.
- **Place any required test orders.** Tests for blood, urine, or imaging may be part of this.
- **Talk about your health concerns and ambitions.** This is an excellent moment to discuss your goals for bettering your health and to ask any questions you may have about it.
- Provide suggestions for your treatment strategy and way of living. Your physician could advise you to make adjustments to your medication, diet, or exercise schedule. If necessary, they might also recommend you to a specialist.

How to get ready for a routine check-in and modification

You can take the following steps to get ready for a routine check-in and adjustment:

- **Jot down any queries you may have.** Making the most of your time with your physician or other healthcare professional will be made easier with this.
- **Enumerate the drugs you take at the moment.** This covers over-the-counter drugs as well as dietary supplements and herbal cures.
- **Bring over any pertinent health records.** Test findings, summaries of hospital discharges, or reports from specialists may be examples of this.
- **Be ready to discuss your issues and goals related to your health.** This is an excellent moment to discuss your goals for bettering your health and to ask any questions you may have about it.

You may make sure that your frequent modifications and check-ins are fruitful and educational by adhering to these suggestions.

Staying Committed to the Pritikin Way

It's critical to keep in mind your initial motivation for beginning the Pritikin Way in order to maintain your commitment. Are you attempting to lower your chance of chronic illnesses, lose weight, or enhance your health? All of these areas have demonstrated the efficacy of the Pritikin Way, so when you find yourself drifting from the path, remind yourself of your objectives.

Integrating the Pritikin Way into your daily routine is a crucial additional piece of advice. It's not something you should think of as an intermittent diet. Rather, concentrate on making long-term, health-conscious decisions. This include maintaining a healthy weight, working out frequently, and controlling stress.

These particular pointers will help you maintain your dedication to the Pritikin Way:

- **Prepare wholesome snacks that you can grab on demand.** This will assist you in steering clear of bad decisions when you're hungry.
- **Make a meal plan in advance.** This will assist you in choosing healthily and preventing impulsive grocery shop purchases.
- **Include exercise in your everyday schedule.** Choose a hobby or pastime that you both like and can fit into your schedule.
- **Locate a safety net.** Having family members or friends who practice the Pritikin Way helps keep you inspired.

- **Take it easy on yourself.** Everyone makes mistakes occasionally. Simply get back up after a setback and try again.

It takes time and work to remain devoted to the Pritikin Way, but the effort is worthwhile. You may lower your risk of chronic diseases, gain weight, and enhance your health with the Pritikin Way.

BREAKFAST

1. AVOCADO TOAST

Equipment

Toaster

Ingredients

- 1 avocado ripe
- 2 slices bread any kind, sourdough is my favorite
- 1 clove garlic cut in half (skin on)
- salt and pepper
- lemon juice optional, from a fresh lemon is best
- extra virgin olive oil good quality

Instructions

1. Halve the avocado and scoop out the pit.

2. To taste, toast the bread.
3. Gently brush the toast's surface with the chopped side of a fresh garlic clove while it's still hot.
4. Using a spoon, remove the avocado flesh and mash it onto the bread using a fork.
5. Add a little salt and pepper.
6. Garnish with olive oil and freshly squeezed lemon juice, or top with chosen toppings. Serve right away.

2. Oatmeal with Berries and Nuts

About the Recipe

136 Calories · 5.8 g Protein · 4.6 g Fiber

Gluten-free

Nut-free

Although they can be produced in a facility that handles gluten, oats do not contain gluten. It's advisable to get oats with a gluten-free label if you have severe sensitivities.

If you have a nut allergy, stay away from adding nuts or milks with nuts as a topping.

INGREDIENTS

Makes Servings

- 1/4 c (20 g) dry rolled oats
- 1/3 c (180 mL) unsweetened low-fat non-dairy milk
- 1/4 c (37 g) blueberries or berries of choice
- 1/4 c (38 g) strawberries or fruit of choice (e.g., banana)

Directions

Follow the directions to prepare the oats. If you'd rather, you can use water in place of the plant milk. You may add any fruit frozen berries, bananas, raisins, or even just bananas.

Nutrition Facts

Calories: 136

Fat: 2.8 g

Saturated Fat: 0.4 g

Calories From Fat: 17.5%

Cholesterol: 0 mg

Protein: 5.8 g

Carbohydrate: 23.4 g

Sugar: 6.2 g

Fiber: 4.6 g

Sodium: 30 mg

Calcium: 119 mg

Iron: 1.4 mg

Vitamin C: 28.2 mg

Beta-Carotene: 15 mcg

Vitamin E: 0.4 mcg

3. Yogurt with Fruit and Granola

INGREDIENTS

- 1/2 cup plain greek yogurt
- 1/4 cup blueberries
- 1/4 cup raspberries
- 1/2 cup cantaloupe
- 1/2 Tbsp goji berries
- 1/2 Tbsp pumpkin seeds
- 1/2 Tbsp sliced almonds
- 1/2 Tbsp coconut shavings
- 1/4 cup granola

INSTRUCTIONS

1. Place the yogurt in a bowl.
2. Add the washed fruit.
3. Top with the seeds, nuts, coconut, and granola.
4. Serve and enjoy

4. EGGS WITH VEGETABLES

INGREDIENTS

- 4 large eggs, lightly beaten

- 1/4 cup fat-free milk

- 1/2 cup chopped green pepper

- 1/4 cup sliced green onions

- 1/4 teaspoon salt

- 1/8 teaspoon pepper

- 1 small tomato, chopped and seeded

Directions

Whisk the eggs and milk together in a small bowl. Add the onions, green pepper, salt, and pepper. Fill a skillet with a little layer of oil. Over medium heat, cook and whisk eggs for 2 to 3 minutes, or until almost set. Add tomato and heat, stirring, until eggs are set through.

Nutrition Facts

3/4 cup: 173 calories, 10g fat (3g saturated fat), 373mg cholesterol, 455mg sodium, 7g carbohydrate (4g sugars, 2g fiber), 15g protein.

Diabetic Exchanges: 2 medium-fat meat, 1 vegetable.

5. SMOOTHIES

INGREDIENTS

(kiwi, banana, blueberries, strawberries, ice, pineapple juice (or orange juice)

ADDITIONS + VARIATIONS

Protein powder is a fantastic method to boost your smoothies' nutritional value and vitamin content.

- chia seeds (high in manganese, phosphorus, copper, iron, magnesium, and calcium)
- flaxseed (high in Vitamin B1, copper, magnesium and phosphorus).

- spinach (high in Vitamin A, Vitamin C, Vitamin K, iron, folate, and potassium)
- kale (high in Vitamin A, Vitamin K, Vitamin B6, Vitamin C, calcium and more!)
- oats (phosphorus, copper, biotin, Vitamin B1)
- Healthy fats that would be good to add include: avocados and nut butters (like almond butter or natural peanut butter).

Change it up by adding

ADDITIONAL FRUITS + VEGGIES: Include your favorites! The selections are unlimited, ranging from leafy greens and various berries to mangoes and pineapples.

SWEETNESS: You can add stevia, vanilla, honey, or a small amount of sugar if you prefer your smoothies to taste a bit sweeter. You can also add sweetness with other sweet fruits.

Dairy and calcium substitutes: Feel free to substitute any preferred type of milk or yogurt. Greek yogurt or even another preferred yogurt flavor are excellent substitutes, as are coconut and almond milk.

SETUP + STORAGE

1. To begin, divide the 5.3 oz of yogurt onto an ice cube tray and place it in the freezer.
2. Cut the bananas into slices and the strawberries into cubes. Transfer them to a baking sheet and freeze.
3. After the yogurt, bananas, and strawberries have frozen, combine them with the mango chunks in a freezer-safe Ziploc bag. Feel free to include any nutritious extras like chia seeds or spinach.
4. For up to three months, FREEZE. When the smoothie is ready, pour the contents of the bag into the blender

along with the ice cubes and almond milk. Mix and savor

LAUNCH

LENTIL SOUP

INGREDIENTS (WITH SUBSTITUTION)

Olive Oil: Avocado oil can be substituted for olive oil.
Onion: You can use a white onion or a yellow onion; both will function well.
Garlic: The best flavor in this case will come from fresh garlic.
Carrots: Make sure the chopped carrots are tiny enough to fit on your spoon together with the other ingredients.

Celery: Before chopping, give your celery a quick rinse under water and pat dry. In this manner, it will be free of any dirt or residue.

Tomatoes: Use diced or crushed tomatoes from a can. Either one will complete the task.

Lentils: Feel free to use either brown or green lentils!

Vegetable Broth: For a less salty taste, use a vegetable broth with low sodium.

Spices: To make this Lentil Soup incredibly flavorful, combine ground cumin, ground coriander, smoked paprika, and a small pinch of salt.

Baby Spinach: To make it easier to take in spoonfuls, slice your spinach into ribbons. Additionally, if you'd like, you can use this instead of kale.

Lemon: Ensure that you are using only freshly squeezed lemon juice never concentrate

How to make lentil soup

- In a big pot, warm the olive oil over medium heat. Add the celery, carrots, onions, and garlic. Cook for about 4–5 minutes, stirring often.

- Add the lentils, vegetable broth, smoked paprika, cumin, and coriander at this point. Also add the can of tomatoes with juices. Mix to combine all the ingredients.

- After bringing to a boil, reduce heat to a simmer, cover, and cook for approximately half an hour, or until lentils are soft and soup has thickened. If desired, mix and thicken slightly using an immersion blender.

- Add the lemon juice and spinach and stir. The spinach will wilt in just a minute or so. Add salt to taste and season.

TUNA SALAD SANDWICH

INGREDIENTS

- Sandwiches made with tuna in oil will taste better than those made with water. Plain oil is not as good as olive oil. But if all you have is tuna in water, then go ahead and push through!

- Different types of canned tuna: Just like most things in life, not all canned tuna is made equal. The price of responsibly harvested and higher-quality tuna is higher.

- Compared to regular, non-whole-egg mayo, which is usually more vinegary and some kinds are, in my opinion, unduly sweet, whole-egg mayo has a smoother flavor. I only have a whole-egg mayo (my favorites are Hellmans and S&W) and Kewpie on hand, both of which are fantastic options!

- Pickles: To add some tang and flavor to the tuna mixture, we're adding both the pickle and the liquid from the jar. Thus, pickle variety is important! I use regular old store-bought dill pickles. Not cornichons, not sweet gherkins, not sour pickles, and not spicy pickles at all!

- (This is just a jest, feel free to use whatever pickles you like. :))

- For freshness, use a green onion. Use baby onions, or eschallots (US: shallots), or 1/4 cup finely chopped red onion in place of the original.

- Celery: To add much-needed crunch, without which the filling would be mushy. chopped finely to blend in.

- Dill: For a fresh, herbaceous taste. My favorite to pair with tuna, though parsley and basil would work just as well.

How to make tuna sandwiches

- Filling for tuna: After draining the oil from the fish, combine it with all the remaining ingredients in a bowl. Break up the tuna into practically a paste-like consistency by using a wooden spoon to mix assertively. It's recommended to mash the pickles and celery to soften the edges and extract some juice for the filling.

- To assemble the sandwich, butter the bread, place two lettuce slices on top, and then add the tuna filling. You can choose how much or how little to use. Place the other bread slip on, then cut and enjoy! For planning ahead, see the note below the picture.

CHICKEN AND AVOCADO WRAP

INGREDIENTS

- 1/2 cup mayonnaise
- 1/2 teaspoon dried basil
- 2 teaspoons lemon juice
- salt and freshly ground black pepper to taste
- 4-5 large flour tortillas
- 2 cups Romaine lettuces , shredded
- 1 avocado , diced
- 5-6 slices bacon , cooked and chopped
- 1 large cooked chicken breast , shredded

Instructions

- Mix the dried basil, lemon juice, mayonnaise, salt, and pepper in a small bowl.
- Combine the shredded lettuce, avocado, bacon, and chicken in a big bowl.
- In a large bowl, add mayonnaise mixture and toss to coat evenly. You may not need to use all of the dressing; just enough to taste.
- Add a generous tablespoon of the filling to each tortilla. Each wrap should be rolled up and, if needed, secured with a toothpick. Have fun!

DINNER

Grilled Salmon with Roasted Vegetables

INGREDIENTS

- 1 medium zucchini, halved lengthwise
- 2 red, orange and/or yellow bell peppers, trimmed, halved and seeded
- 1 medium red onion, cut into 1-inch wedges
- 1 tablespoon extra-virgin olive oil
- ½ teaspoon salt, divided
- ½ teaspoon ground pepper
- 1 ¼ pounds salmon fillet, cut into 4 portions
- ¼ cup thinly sliced fresh basil
- 1 lemon, cut into 4 wedges

Directions

1. Grill on medium-high heat.

2. After applying oil to the zucchini, peppers, and onion, season with 1/4 teaspoon salt. Add pepper and the remaining 1/4 teaspoon of salt to the salmon.

3. Arrange the vegetables and salmon slices on the grill with the skin side down. Cook the vegetables for 4 to 6 minutes on each side, turning them once or twice, or until they are just soft and have grill marks. Fry the salmon for 8 to 10 minutes, or until it flakes when examined with a fork, without flipping it.

4. Once the vegetables have cooled down sufficiently, roughly chop them and combine them in a big bowl. If preferred, remove the skin from the salmon fillets and serve with the veggies. Serve each dish with a lemon wedge and garnish with one tablespoon of basil.

INGREDIENTS

Lentils

- ½ cup dry lentils (French green lentils or regular brown lentils), or 1 ½ cups cooked lentils (leftover or from a can, rinsed and drained)
- 1 bay leaf
- 1 large garlic clove, peeled but left whole
- ¼ teaspoon salt
- 2 cups vegetable broth or water

Everything else

- 2 cups marinara sauce
- 8 ounces whole-grain pasta (or 12 ounces, if you like your pasta less spicy than mine)
- Optional garnishes: grated Parmesan or vegan Parmesan and/or chopped fresh basi

DIRECTIONS

1. Before cooking the lentils, rinse them in a fine-mesh colander and sort through them for debris (I once bit into a little rock). Combine the lentils, broth, garlic, bay leaf, and salt in a small saucepan.
2. Over medium-high heat, bring the mixture to a simmer; then, lower the heat to maintain a low simmer. Depending on the age and variety of the lentils, simmering will take 20 to 35 minutes or longer until the lentils are soft and cooked thoroughly. After draining the lentils and throwing away the garlic and bay leaf, cover the saucepan and leave it there.
3. In the interim, heat up a big pot of salted water to a boil. Follow the instructions on the package to cook the pasta until it's al dente. After draining, put the pasta back in the pot and reserve.
4. Warm the lentils and marinara together over a medium heat, stirring to combine. Pasta should be divided into bowls. Warm marinara and lentils could be topped with Parmesan cheese and/or chopped fresh basil, if desired. Warm up and serve. When covered

and kept in the refrigerator, leftovers can last
for up to four days.

CONCLUSION: EMBRACING A HEALTHIER FUTURE

Accepting a healthy future is a process rather than an end goal. It involves gradually implementing tiny, long-lasting adjustments to your food, exercise regimen, and way of life. Here are some pointers to get you going:

1. Begin by defining reasonable objectives. Avoid making drastic changes too soon as this will only make you give up and become discouraged. Focus on implementing one tiny adjustment at a time instead. For instance, you may begin by including a serving of vegetables in every meal or by going for three weekly walks of thirty minutes each. Once those adjustments are mastered, you can move on to other objectives.

2. Look for wholesome meals that you like consuming. Trying to make oneself consume nutritious things you don't enjoy is pointless. Finding nutritious substitutes for the items you enjoy eating is the key. For instance, consider baked chicken or fish in instead of fried chicken. Consider quinoa or brown rice in place of white rice. Try sparkling water, unsweetened tea, or water in place of sugary beverages.

3. Add fun to working out. Your likelihood of sticking with a fitness regimen decreases if you don't love it. Look for hobbies or pastimes that suit your lifestyle. Try swimming, bicycling, or dancing, for instance, if you're not a fan of running. If you're limited on time, consider dividing your workouts into shorter bursts over the day.

4. Get adequate rest. Getting enough sleep is critical to general health and wellbeing. Get seven to eight hours of sleep every night.

5. Resolve tension. Unhealthy eating patterns, weight gain, and other health issues can be brought on by stress. Look for stress-reduction techniques that are beneficial, like yoga, meditation, or exercise.

6. Be in the company of upbeat people. Your social circle can greatly influence your health-related behaviors. Make sure everyone around you encourage you to pursue your dreams and give you confidence in yourself.

Though it's not always simple, embracing a healthier future is worthwhile. You'll have more energy, feel better about yourself, and have a lower risk of developing chronic diseases when you make smart decisions.

Here are some more pointers to assist you in welcoming a healthier future:

- **Learn for yourself.** Making healthy decisions will be simpler the more you understand about leading a healthy lifestyle. Examine publications on stress reduction, physical activity, and diet. For tailored counsel, speak with your physician or a certified dietician.
- **Have patience.** Making changes to your lifestyle and habits takes time. If you don't notice results right away, don't give up. Simply keep going and make wise decisions.
- **Honor your accomplishments.** Spend some time celebrating your accomplishments when you reach your goals. This will support your continued motivation and onward motion.
- **Accepting a healthy future is an ongoing process.** However, you can enhance your quality of life, well-being, and health by implementing modest but long-lasting adjustments.